THE SEDUCTIVE PINK CRYSTAL

By

Isaac Alexis M.D.

Acknowledgements

First, I want to thank My Lord and Savior Jesus Christ for the privilege of taking care of these precious souls that have a Substance Use Disorder. It has taught me to be Christ's Arms extended and to him I am eternally grateful. I also Thank the Patient's personally that I have had the privilege of taking care of with various Addictions.

I also want to take the time to invite those who don't know Jesus as Lord and Savior to Confess him as Savior of your LIFE and accept him into your heart. It will be the BEST decision you have made in your LIFE. Romans 10:9 that if thou shalt confess with thy mouth the Lord Jesus, and shall believe in thine heart that God have raised him from the dead, thou shall be saved.

To Sanja Gumbar thanks for your wonderful

Cover Design for this book which has meant so much to me.

To My very patient Wife and children Alvera, Praise & Isaac as I missed many basketball games to write this book I truly thank you for your patience and love you.

To My Mom and Dad thanks for giving me Life.

To Dr. A. McDermott thanks for being my Inspiration for studying Neuroscience for the past 20 Years at Columbia University.

Thanks Lightning Press for wonderful Print Renditions of this my Most Precious Literary Work.

Last but not least in memory of my Cousin who Died from a Drug Overdose - You will NEVER, EVER, EVER, EVER be forgotten as I think of you EVERY NIGHT and DAY.

Introduction

What do you think when you hear of a crystal? You probably think of some beautiful gem like a Red Beryl that retails at $10,000 per carat or opals that come for around $2,300 per carat. These are certainly beautiful crystals that would make you get you in the good books of your girlfriend again, after you have had a heated argument with her. Crystals go back to the times of the ancient Egyptians, who buried their dead with a quartz on their foreheads. This was thought to guide the recently deceased safely into the afterlife. Unlike the Egyptians, the Ancient Greeks believed that before entering battle, if soldiers crushed hematite and rubbed it on their bodies, this would make them indestructible. Hematite on the OUTSIDE is metallic silver to black in color but when rubbed on a surface, it leaves a red streak! Do not judge a book by its cover, I guess. In industry, hematite is used for producing pigments and for radiation shields.

Crystals are also used in solar cells. These same solar cells are utilized to power things ranging from calculators to space vehicles. Transistors use crystals to regulate subatomic particle flows that detect and amplify radio signals and act like digital switches. Transistor radios are such an example. There are liquid crystals that are used for heat, magnetism, and mechanics in the world of physics and engineering. Common uses for liquid crystals would be in pocket calculators. In New Age medicinal practices, amethyst is used to treat cephalgia (headache in layman's terms). Aquamarine regulates the immune system, the cardiovascular system, and the lymph nodes. Carnelian is supposed to help with energy, the reproductive system, and menstrual cramps. Citrine is supposed to cleanse the spleen, kidneys, and liver. Coral is for aiding in metabolism, the spine, and tissue regeneration. Emeralds are to help with the thymus and childbirth, and jade is supposed to cleanse the blood and nervous system. Rubies are to help with cholesterol and blood clots. Sapphire helps with inflammation, fevers, tuberculosis, and nosebleeds. In Daniel 10:6, we read about the Most High God: “His body also was like the beryl, and his face as the appearance of lightning, and his eyes as lamps of fire, and his arms and his feet like in colour to polished brass, and the voice of his words like the voice of a multitude.”

Let us go back to the beryl for a moment. The Red Beryl in its most refined form is over $10,000 a carat! Wow! That is a lot of money for sure. The word “crystal” comes from the Greek word *krustullos*, which means ice. In ancient times, cultures believed that crystals were the eternal ice from the heavens. In India, in Ayurvedic medicine, crystals have healing properties. In Roman culture, they had amulets made from various crystals to attract health, fortune, and success in battle just like the Greeks. We see from the above descriptions of crystals that they generally benefit the human race, or at least should have that effect for us to be interested in them in the first place. Well, we will now look at another crystal that is not so BENIGN to human beings or their lives and, in fact, is very detrimental and known as the Pink Crystal.

Table of Contents

Chapter One

Homeboy Can Run!

We will now delve more deeply into exactly what my cousin Susan was most addicted to and, yes, HINT, HINT, what I mentioned in my first book, “Life and Death behind the Brick and Razor—Code Red Diamond.” She grew up in Brooklyn, New York, in the 1980s. She had a $300+ a day habit and stole continuously from my Aunt Claire to support her habit. She was also very quiet and did not speak much. She would leave the house at midnight and not return until 7 the next morning.

Once, I was at my aunt’s in Brooklyn and suddenly heard gunshots. My Aunt Claire called out loudly, “Susan, Susan! Where are you?” There was no response from Susan. I was saying a quick and quiet prayer for her safety. While sending up this quick prayer for her, I peered out of the corner of my eye from the front window to the first floor, where I saw some youths with a ziplock bag (gallon size) and the cops in hot pursuit on foot, running with all their might. Just watching them was amazing. The young guys were clearing those red and yellow fences like they were hurdles at some 1984 Olympic track and field event. The youths ran in their green high-top Pro-Keds basketball sneakers for about 500 feet and then threw this ziplock bag on the ground while still running. It was amazing to see them run with their jeans down to almost their kneecaps, but boy could they run. Anyway, one of the youths stood at about six foot one and was bald, and the other had a flattop haircut and stood at five foot ten and was very quick on his feet, easily clearing each one of those red and yellow fences. The cops said, “Freeze and put your hands up now!” The first cop was still rigorously pursuing the young men by foot, while the second cop, quite winded from the pursuit, stopped and scooped up the evidence in his right hand. I could hear them clearly. The first cop asked the second, "What is it?" The second cop answered, "I don't know but it looks like crystal!" The first cop asked, "What color is it?" The second responded, "It looks like it has a red, maybe even pink, color, man!" The first cop then asked, "How many rocks in there, man?" To which the second cop responded, "Looks like 12 or 13!" The first cop said, "Yep, they're going to do some serious hard time for this!"

The first cop was around 45 years old and stood at around six foot four, and the second cop was much younger, around 21 years old and stood at around five foot six. The first cop told the second, "We will analyze this pink crystal."

The first cop finally caught up with the two fleeing youths, placed them in handcuffs, and asked them frankly, "Guys, I'm gonna give you one chance and one chance only to answer my question! What's in the bag?" He was in plainclothes, sporting black Levi jeans, a white T-shirt, and white Adidas sneakers, and was running out of breath and sweating profusely. He had a certain swagger when he walked, like he was saying to the world: there are not going to be any drugs sold on my watch.

The second cop wore a navy-blue T-shirt, black Lee jeans, and suede blue Adidas sneakers. Back in the day when you wore Adidas sneakers, you were instantly in the cool crowd. I remember having my first blue suede pair, and the kids in elementary school who normally ignored me would all of a sudden notice me and sit with me in the cafeteria as we exchanged comic books with one another. One kid named Derrick would always tell me, "Yo, Zac, your clothes were once in style... in the age of the dinosaurs!" After this cold and cutting remark, I felt my face turn beet red and sweat all of a sudden pour down my face. I answered, "I'm not really into clothes, man." Looking at his grade point average and mine, you could tell who studied harder and who dressed to impress—with grades not necessarily being the highest priority. Derrick would look at the soles of my sneakers when I walked and would say, “Man, Zac, those sneakers are so thin on the bottom I thought you wore them as soon as you were born!” I would respond, “Very funny, man!”

I knew something about Derrick that he did not know I knew! Even though he wore the latest sneakers to school, during class I would see him take off both his sneakers and socks and scratch his feet violently and with such ferocity that flakes from the outer layers of his feet would pile up on the cold green vinyl composition tile. Scratch, scratch, scratch—this would go on for at least ten minutes at a time and create, in the process, a miniature mountain of white flakes on the green tiled floor. Sometimes his foot would bleed, and the red blood on top of the pile of white flakes, which itself was supported by the green tile, looked like a Christmas tree that a Smurf could enjoy.

But the stench from his foot was another matter. It nearly knocked me out on one occasion, and Ms. Smith, our Social Studies teacher, blurted out during the middle of a lesson, “What is that awful smell?” Now, Ms. Smith was a no-nonsense type of teacher. If you blurted out an answer to her question without first raising your hand, she would make you write 500 times, “I Will Not Speak Out of Turn and Must First Raise My Hand.” She was an intense teacher. She came from South Carolina and had a sweet and warm, congenial Southern accent. But if you were one of her students that DARED to talk out of turn, which meant speaking without raising your hand, that warm nature that used to embrace you would then suddenly drop you to the floor and spit lava-hot grits and butter into your eyeballs, setting them ablaze as you took those lava-hot eyes and fixed them forward to where Ms. Smith was writing your name on the board as part of the list of hooligans that were going to spend time in HARD

TIME—detention—for two hours.

Anyway, Ms. Smith said, “I want to know what is that foul smell!” I found tears slowly forming in my eyes as often happens when I’m about to burst into laughter but trying to hold it in. I wanted so desperately to reveal the location of this funk that was sitting right next to me. I looked into Derrick’s eyes and he could tell I’d been laughing. He gave me the stare of death and muttered, “If you tell Ms. Smith it’s me, I’m gonna jump you after school!”

So, Ms. Smith gave all of us the ultimatum: “If none of you wants to confess, how would ALL OF YOU like doing detention for two hours after school today?” There was no way in perdition I was going to do two hours of hard time with Principal Wallace. Principal Wallace stood at nearly seven feet tall and his hands were so big he could not only palm a basketball, he could hold it as if it was a mere golf ball! This man just scared the life out of me.

There was no way I was going to serve my sentence of two hours doing hard time under Principal Wallace's supervision in the Home Economics office. That room was small with a musty odor and had a dreary slate-to-pewter color composition to it. And on top of that, being with Derrick and his funky feet would be intolerable. That was torture. He could kick my butt all he wanted, I thought, but I was not doing detention for this guy! I made up in my mind that I was going to sanitize the situation.

I raised my hand high. I heard Derrick mutter under his breath, "If you tell her it's me, you gonna be beat bad!" To which I replied, "Man, your feet just stink so bad and I'm doing this for survival!" What I was trying to survive was the noxious injury his horrific feet were causing to the lining of my lungs. On a bad day, his feet smelled like ammonia and I could literally feel my nose burning. I often thought the hairs from my nose also were falling out from the horrific stench that was housed in those sneakers of his. Ms. Smith said, “Isaac, what is it?” I replied, “I know where the stench is coming from!!” She replied, “OK., so where, Isaac, do you think it’s coming from?” I replied, “Today is Tuesday and across the hall is the Home Economics class where they teach us how to cook!” Ms. Smith looked at me, seemingly not too impressed. She responded, “Isaac, if you are wasting my time and preventing your fellow classmates from getting an education, I’ll personally see to it that you do three hours of detention!” She continued, “Do I make myself clear, young man?” I responded, “Yes, ma’am!” So Ms. Smith continued, “You think that the Home Economics class has something to do with it?” “Yes, ma’am,” I responded, careful not to anger this woman who was close friends with Principal Wallace. The Home Economics class was terrible at emptying the garbage outside after they finished class there. One time, they had been making sardine pizzas and forgot to throw out the 20 or so sardine cans and two dozen eggs from their class garbage, and it stunk up our Social Studies class for one week! I reminded Ms. Smith of this incident, and she bluntly responded, “I suppose you have a point!” She continued, “I’m going to go next door and see if that is the case, but if it’s not, ALL of y’all are going to do detention.”

She walked 25 feet across the hall and opened the door of the Home Economics class and, sure enough, she uttered a tear-wrenching scream, “Ahhhhhhhhhh!!!!” I ran from my chair with lightning speed and pushed those Adidas on my feet to their absolute limits in order to come to her side in a heartbeat! Words cannot begin to describe the pile of garbage I saw in that Home Economics garbage pail. There were at least 30 empty egg shells, ten rotting banana peels, 25 cans of empty sardines, and two dead rats with massive beige-colored maggots eating the rat carcasses on top of that putrescent dump.

You really needed a gas mask to enter that room—which smelled like hydrogen sulfide. “Let’s get out of here now!” Ms. Smith struggled to get out of her mouth. I could see from the corner of my eyes that her lips were twitching and both of her hands were tightly clenched. It appeared those long pink nails of Ms. Smith were about to cut right into her palms. I said, “Ms. Smith, what’s the matter?” She replied, “My stomach hurts.” I could tell she was doing everything in her power not to vomit.

We finally came from behind the enemy lines of the fetid Home Economics classroom and were back in the safe domain of our Social Studies classroom. Ms. Smith then announced to the class, “You kids are lucky. Had it not been for Isaac letting me know where that foul smell was coming from, all of y’all would have been in detention for two hours come 3 o’clock today!” Ms. Smith continued, “I’m going to make sure that Mr. Finch gets a stern warning from Principal Wallace for keeping such a nasty classroom!"

Despite being a strict disciplinarian, Ms. Smith dressed like a model. She always enjoyed shopping at Barneys New York, and this day was adorned in an osman gray poncho-style satin blouse with Prada floral slim crop pants in beige and, to top it all off, had the most elegant Ryan Roche white cashmere silk oversized long cardigan sweater. Ms. Smith sported an ombre lob hairstyle that was simply mesmerizing.

Anyway, Mr. Finch was extremely relaxed and often forgot things—things that were important! I remember it was a parent-teacher conference once and he forgot to show up! It took several calls from Principal Wallace to Mr. Finch to finally get him to the school to meet with the parents and, to top it off, he forgot the files for each student that he was supposed to give the parents an update on. My mother remarked one time, "What is this man doing?" Mom continued, "When I ask him specific questions about you academically, all he says is you are good and listen intently." I could see mom getting frustrated, but she just said, "Let's just see the next teacher on your list!" To which I simply responded, "Sounds very good indeed!"

Anyway, after coming back from the wastelands of that empty Home Economics classroom, I saw Derrick still scratching that darn foot of his! What he needed was some athlete's foot cream! I was tired of those flakes accumulating on the floor. As I sat down, Derrick gave me this half grin and said, "Boy, you sure lucky, man. I thought you was dumb enough to be the teacher's pet and squeal on me, for which I would have had to kick your butt!" To which I responded, "Derrick, your feet stink. Put your socks and sneakers on!" The type of floors I felt that school needed especially for Derrick's funky feet were Flotex. Flotex is easy to care for and maintains a high antimicrobial environment after it is sanitized, and is dust mite-prohibitive, so it is great for people with allergies.

Anyway, both of those cops dressed pretty HIP—and you would have thought that they shopped at V.I.M. The youths looked in the bag and then at the cop and simultaneously declared, “Yo, Mr. 5-0, we don’t know!” “There are people above us that hand this stuff to us who are pretty mean and we just don’t ask questions!” the youths continued. The first cop then screamed, “Somehow I don’t believe you!” He declared, “Well, it’s too bad because tonight the two of you are going to get booked, and in the morning, you will get such a tough sentence from the judge that you will be lucky if you are out in time to collect Social Security in your sixties!” One of the youths responded, “You can’t talk to us like that, man!” The first cop responded confidently, “So, what are you going to do about it?” The youth responded, “Take me out of these cuffs and I’ll show you what I’ll do!” The second cop tried to control himself but burst out laughing at the youth's reply. The first cop responded with a thunderous, "Shut your mouth now!" And he went on to tell his partner, "Brother, you can't be laughing at these idiots—it just encourages them that much more!" The second cop responded, "Sorry, it just came out." The cops placed the youths in their 1977 blue Plymouth Fury squad car and drove off with lights flashing on top of the vehicle as it cruised down Atlantic Avenue and turned onto Troy Avenue. I have seen many of those 1977 Plymouth Furys thunder down Liberty Avenue, sirens blasting after gunfights with youths assuming the best way to assert their street toughness. and hence credibility, was to pull a Smith & Wesson Model 29 on each other quickly and decisively, leading to many fatalities in South Jamaica, Queens. Those gun battles were often over a girl, but many, many times were turf wars over drugs. I saw in the parks guys slyly looking over their shoulder and passing small bags to each other in whispered tones. Then an unmarked cop car would often burst on the scene, turn on those classic blue and white lights, and you'd see five guys shout, "Yo, bail out, bail out. The 5-0 gonna get you!" For those of you who do not know the street lingo, 5-0 refers to police officers or any member of the law enforcement community. The term came from the classic *Hawaii Five-0* TV show from the 1960s.

Anyway, my aunt called Susan again and then finally got a response from her: "I'm upstairs in my bedroom sleeping and you woke me up, Ma!" I would rather have my cousin safe inside the comfort of this Brooklyn brownstone than outside on those dangerous streets! There we were as a family at Thanksgiving dinner eating a savory meal of Trinidad spiced chicken with okra, oxtail soup and lentil soup, callaloo (a West Indian type of spinach), candied yams with coconut flavored rice, and black beans. I was chewing the food so fast as it was so tasty that I forgot that my aunt had just taken everything fresh off the stove and out of the oven! I must not have noticed the steam profusely rising to her ceiling from the food as it came straight out of the oven—I burned nearly two-thirds of my tongue gulping that food down without swallowing. I rushed to the bathroom to gulp down some ice-cold water under the gushing faucet. Aunt Claire had such a neat home and her Kohl faucets were something out of a 5-star Hotel Intercontinental. The ice-cold water of Brooklyn, New York, was refreshing coming out of that Brownstone edifice. If you could bottle this stuff, you could open up your own bootleg company and be a friggin' millionaire overnight. My mom said irately, "Ike, what are you up to?" She continued, "You know it's rude to leave the table without saying excuse me." I retorted, "But Ma, my tongue was on fire and it hurt badly." (The average human tongue has as many as 10,000 taste buds, and that number dwindles by around

30% to 40% as we age. I thought that I had burned a good number of those taste buds, as I could not taste for a while after that incident.) After thoroughly explaining my scar to my mother like an attorney talking to the judge in court, she responded, “That’s nothing compared to how hot your other end is gonna be if you don’t start showing some manners when you’re out in public!” “Yes, Ma” was my simple response to her. I wasn’t about to anger this madwoman with samurai sword-like reflexes. If you were dumb enough to blink even for one second and you accidentally broke one of her endless bylaws or crossed in front of her while she was walking, you could kiss goodbye to the privilege of sitting down for the next two weeks, as your ass would remind you each time you sat down that maybe that wasn’t the wisest thing to do because your rear quarters were beaten raw from the minor violation committed two weeks prior. It was similar to a payday. I knew dad’s payday was every two weeks because I seemed to commit one of these violations, irritating my mom about once every two weeks, and that is the exact amount of time it would take for my behind to cool back down again! Two weeks was my relief period. I would get my allowance from dad—a fat $2.50 for all the backbreaking labor I did like cleaning the dirty muddy basement and vacuuming my parents' cars and raking leaves among, other things.

Anyway, back to the dinner at Aunt Claire's house… After cooling my tongue off with that ice-cold delicious mineral water, I passed Susan, who was sitting on her bed. She was quiet, and I thought it was extremely weird that she wasn't eating with the rest of us. Who in the world would not eat Aunt Claire's food? It was the best in all of Brooklyn. She was told continuously that she should open her own restaurant, and I truly agreed with that assessment. She cooked even better than my dad, and he was a world-class cook in the preparation of Trinidad-stylechicken dishes. Aunt Claire saved a lot on contractor work on her ceilings and drywall repair, as all the workers wanted as pay was her delicious meals! I'm dead serious! No one could resist the allure of her tempting meals. I would get a $20 bill as a Christmas present from Aunt Claire, which at my age was like hitting the jackpot, but all I wanted was her chicken and rice. I could eat that 24/7/365.

Aunt Claire wore a gentle smile and was like a rose in motion. She could not harm a mosquito even if she wanted to. Her voice was like canary's singing in all its majestic glory on a splendid spring day. She had that gentle disposition from Grandpa Alexis back in Trinidad. Had Granpops been alive today, he would have been 110 years old. God bless his soul in heaven. Aunt Claire always encouraged me to study hard and avoid bad influences at all costs! She was my father's older sister and the eldest of 13 brothers and sisters.

So, as I passed Susan's room, I noticed that she didn't want to make eye contact. Her room had three-inch thick plush beige safavieh carpet and was a warm place where the love of my aunt for her daughter was simply palpable. The carpet made a neat rectangle around ten feet by twelve feet. Once you stepped on this carpet, it was as if you were walking on a piece of cloud 50,000 feet overhead. This carpet was the stuff that kings and queens would walk on. I had this callous on my left big toe on the lateral edge, and guess where I would walk first thing when coming into Aunt Claire's home? You guessed it! I would walk on that safavieh plush carpet and it was as if I were walking on clouds of cotton. The pleasure of stepping on that carpet would sort of give me a head rush—it felt so good! Susan's room was painted a relaxing off-brown color similar to an umber hue. It was gentle on the eye and didn't blind you in any way like some rooms do when the lights are on. The painting was done once a year at Aunt Claire's home as she was extremely meticulous. "Don't let her calm demeanor fool you," my dad would go on. She works hard and at her job as an Administrative Executive, but when she comes home, that is when the work truly begins. Aunt Claire could be seen scrubbing the corners of the walls making sure all stains, spider webs, and so forth were cleaned before any guests ever came by. The chandelier that adorned Susan's room was splendid. It was a crystal chandelier with the crystals delicately hanging downward, effortlessly working with the effects of gravity, with the eight lights standing at attention like confident soldiers about to go into battle. Anyway, grand chandeliers were a recurrent motif in Aunt Claire's home. It was like stepping into a palace whenever I came by to visit. The wood bureaus and desks looked like furniture out of the Oval Office.

Now, I decided that I would initiate the conversation. "Susan, why don't you want to eat?" To which she responded, "I'm not hungry!" She gave me, at that time, a deep penetrating stare as if to say buzz off! She might have been an older cousin, but I would not be scared so easily. I then responded, "Come and join us at the dinner table!" "No, I don't feel like it and I ain't hungry!" she replied. Susan was skin and bones, and at that time, I did not know there were other issues at play. "Susan, how could you not eat your own mom's food?" I asked incredulously. "I just don't want any," Susan again responded firmly.

I just shrugged my shoulders and resumed my walk to the table that would have my feast awaiting. I ate for the next two hours until my belly made me look as if I had ingested a planetary body. I could have thought that my belly was so big that the moon was closer to the horizon than usual. I could have believed that it was from the gravitational effects exerted by my belly on the surrounding cosmos!

Susan's was an interesting case, and I asked my Aunt Claire why she wouldn't eat any food, and Auntie said it was a long story. My dad intervened and said, "Son, I'll My mom was less pleased and let me know with her ice-cold stare that I could be in for one of her judicial hearings that would have only one verdict: a two weeker. As in, speak another word and your gluteus maximus will be burning from a leather strapping on your backside, which should recover in about two weeks! I decided to let reason and common sense take over, so I shut my mouth and did not utter another word, and hence, my backside was saved and it profusely thanked me!

As I climbed into the back of my dad's 1978 Ford LTD, I knew that I would get this mystery solved. I pondered what my next move would be to strategically find out from dad what Susan's problem was. I knew there had to be an answer to why Susan, who used to be more outgoing and also used to weigh 150 pounds at five foot four, now weighed only 103 pounds! What the heck was going on here? Something was just not adding up! And I would find out! I considered all these thoughts in the back of my dad's classic car.

That car had a relaxing color to it and was a mix between cobalt blue and an Oxford blue. It was a two-door man cave on four smooth Michelin tires that felt like you were riding on a carpet flying effortlessly on the wind. I see why my mom liked dad when they started dating. With wheels as cool as this, you could not get any better with shining chrome rims. I could wake up and brush my teeth using those four sparkling chrome rims as my mirror. That 4.9-liter engine roared whenever my dad pressed on the gas. Even though the production years were from 1969 to 1978, it was still cooler than a modern-day Lamborghini Aventador V-12 engine. I would take a fully tuned-up vintage 1978 Ford LTD over a Lambho any day! That’s my story and, yes, I’m sticking to it! The kids in the neighborhood would say to me, “Yo, Isaac, is that your dad’s car?!” “Of course,” I would shout. Who did they think it belonged to—Casper the Friendly Ghost? It was so attractive that it got stolen several times at my dad’s job in Brooklyn!

That’s when dad would call mom and let her know the bad news. “Honey,” my dad would begin. “What is it, Alex?” she responded. To which he replied, “Someone stole the car.” “Is that the only time you care to call me?” she barked angrily. “Can’t you at least call to say ‘I love you’ or something romantic?” she said. She continued, “You put your hands on that car and touch it delicately more often than you do me!” She continued, “You don’t even ask me what my dreams or hopes or desires are!” To which he responded, “You gonna pick me up or what?” “Ok, punk, I’ll get you, but you gonna treat me to some chocolates on the way home. I’m tired of this bull!" she responded.

So, it was off in the Emerald Green 1975 Mercury Comet. If you thought your car was small, my dear brothers and sisters, you have not seen anything yet or rather I should say, you have not felt anything yet. That car was so small that all you had to do was sneeze in the back seat and you'd sustain a concussion from your head hitting the front windshield—or at least it felt like that! If you accidentally dropped your handkerchief in that vehicle, you'd automatically have wall-to-wall plush carpeting.

One time a Chihuahua with a smooth silky black and mahogany coat accidentally jumped into that emerald green Comet, and one of my friends that just happened to be passing by said, "Yo, Zac, I didn't know you had a Rottweiler!" James always had dogs of all types—Pit Bull, German shepherd, Rottweiler—and was one of the cool cats of the hood. Standing at a muscular six foot two at the age of 12, he was someone no one dared mess with.

He knew some Hapkido martial arts, so if you ever thought of fighting him, he would tie you up into a pretzel before you could even think of sucker punching him! I said to James that this was not a Rottweiler, so he came closer to look at what exactly I was talking about. He was no more than 50 feet across the street and when he came closer he said, "Oh, snap, man, your ride is so small that I thought that your dog was a Rott!" James continued, "I didn't know that it was a Chihuahua!" I knew my mom's car was exquisitely small, but I was thinking to myself at this point, "James, maybe I can direct you to a good optometrist!" Even if James needed glasses, he would not use them. To wear glasses in the hood was so uncool that James would risk getting hit by the Q-17 bus before donning those circular windows on his nose—as he referred to what kids with glasses wore.

One time, Shaka, the neighborhood bully that knocked kids' glasses off their face, had a confrontation with

James. Shaka was a lanky six foot four kid. He wore black Lee jeans and a white tank top. He would hang out at the 179 Street subway station in Jamaica, Queens. Shaka ran up behind this kid who stood at five feet three and slapped the glasses off the boy. Little did Shaka know that James was watching from across the street near the local Burger King. James always loved downing a juicy Whopper and a Coke. Those Whoppers were huge and were the size of dinner plates back in the day. When James saw this felony being committed by the neighborhood tough, he did one thing. He dropped his burger and told Shaka, "You gonna tell that small kid sorry and pick up his glasses for him, man!" Shaka laughed loud and hard. "Man, you crazy" he retorted. Shaka continued, "If you don't get out of my face, Little Butterfly, you gonna be fortunate to pick up the piece of face I'm gonna slam to the ground!"

Up to that point, my favorite butterfly was the Monarch

butterfly. This butterfly migrates all the way from parts of Canada and the Northeastern United States to the Sierra Sanctuary in Mexico, some 3,000 miles away! Amazing! By the way, the other name for the Monarch butterfly is the "Common Tiger." Little did Shaka know what he was calling James every time he said "Butterfly." James continued in a calm voice, "Shaka, pick up them glasses and give them to that kid!" Shaka said, "Little Butterfly, you ain't crap!" Shaka did not realize James was a second-degree black belt in Hapkido and that he was in for a good butt-slamming!

Shaka then got up in James's face and looked down on him. They were now face-to-face, and by this time, a crowd of around 50 people had slowly gathered. The small kid who was the main character in all of this was sweating and teary-eyed. Shaka continued to taunt James by moving another inch closer to his face. Shaka had a broad grin on his face as he must have called James

"Butterfly" at least 15 times! One person from the crowd shouted, "James, you gonna let that punk Shaka talk to you like that?" Shaka answered the man in the crowd, "There ain't nothing this coward is going to do about it!" But Shaka did not know that James was slowly forming a fist with his right hand. The left hand very, very slowly followed. The crowd that was initially bustling in anticipation was about to get their money's worth. Shaka was about to say "Butterfly" for the sixteenth time. But "Butter—" was all he could get out before James threw a ferocious right uppercut, then followed it with a left hook across Shaka's chiseled mandible. This was the followed with a 540-degree Taekwondo kick delivered intricately well to the left posterior ear all within seconds of each other. Shaka's white tank top was now a drenched crimson red as Shaka was slammed to the ground—knocked out. James continued, "Let me tell all of you guys in the neighborhood, 'You ain't messing with the little kids!'" He continued, "These little kids can't defend themselves and they sure can't help it if their eyes are weak!" The crowd had dropped their jaws in amazement, and then without uttering a word, they walked away. James, the Neighborhood Cool Guy with the New Dogs, was now transformed into James, the Neighborhood Enforcer—or should I say "The Common Tiger"!

James stood over Shaka, looking down on him, and then took the lid off of his forty-eight-ounce Cola and threw it across Shaka's face, jolting him out of his comatose-like state. Shaka had this beard that was at least three inches thick but now was caked in blood. James began, "Now, Shaka, I'm gonna do the talkin." James continued, "Pick up the kid's glassesnow—or else!" This time, without saying a word, Shaka picked up the glasses and handed it them to the small kid. James continued, "I'd better never see you picking trouble with any kid ever again!" Shaka held his head low and walked away. His crimson-stained white tank top was now transformed to a garnet colored hue.

James walked the little boy all the way home, which was another 1,000 feet ahead. I wanted to have moves like that in a fight! I knew no one would bother me if I possessed such moves. The way James could combine punches and kicks was effortless and orchestrated like a conductor of the New York Philharmonic. It was skilled fighting at its finest. The Common Tiger was decades ahead of the MMA venues in Las Vegas. James was seven years older than me, but he seemed to possess a father-like attitude when it came to protecting the smaller kids.

While most older dudes would think it cool to push a smaller kid down on the grass to impress their girlfriend, James would have none of that. James dated military girls that were very disciplined and were very strong and independent women. I would hear him talk with Terry, his girl from the army, and she would inform him that he needed to work hard and challenge himself mentally, physically, and spiritually to push through his natural limits and never accept defeat in anything he did. "James, being tired is NEVER an option!" Terry firmly stated. I thought, does she know who she is talking to? This Common Tiger is a second-degree black belt in martial arts! James's first love was his music, and he could turn it on or off whenever he pleased with the flick of his wrist. He could not do this with Terry. She was one tough sister. "All you do is listen to your music!" screamed Terry. "You don't even look me in the eye when I'm talking to you!" she continued. "I only have a week off from the base and you hold that radio more than you do me! "Beneath that tough exterior, Terry possessed a gentle, passionate soul of a woman—the kind that liked poetry being read to her in Central Park while being fed Godiva dark chocolates with raspberry filling. Terry stood at six feet tall and had a curvaceous figure. Her face was a smooth beige composition without a wrinkle in it. She walked tall and erect, and those soft brown eyes and braided wavy black hair were a wonderful sight to behold. I would see them hold hands and laugh in each other's company, but I knew a key element was missing. James began, "Terry...Baby, you know I care for you." She responded, "There you go again, James. You can't even say the word!" James went on, "I have no idea, baby, what you are saying." Terry began, "Not once have you said those three words to me for the 18 months we been together!" James looked at her and said, "You mean, 'Please hug me?'" She threw a ferocious stare in his direction and said, "No dumb dumb, 'I Love You!'" Terry continued, "What's wrong with you guys? You all act as if you are going to lose your manhood if you say those three simple words. I don't know if I want to be with somebody that cannot simply express how they genuinely feel in this relationship."

The next time I saw James he had a Sony boom box radio in one hand playing the latest rap music beats while walking a Doberman dog with the other hand. It appeared that he was single again and Terry had left him. Anyway his dog was even hip, running those four legs to the exact beat of the bass drums of the song. James's favorite boom box stereo was the Panasonic RX-5080 AM/FM cassette player. He would blast his boom box at at least 100 decibels and you would feel your heart thumping in your chest as scores of bass drums all in unison reached deafening crescendos. It was as if those drums fed off of each other. The drums best sounded like the djembe drums of West Africa where the purpose of the drum was for everyone to gather in peace. But the way James blasted that boom box, it sounded like a war between him and the other guys in the neighborhood, who would have boom box duels to see who had the most dominating stereo boom box within a five-block radius. From the last word on the street James was the Dominating King. However, there were some colonels, majors, and captains that were closing in on James's Musical Hierarchy. James would also change cool dogs as quickly as he would change radio stations one after another, like a pair of socks changed after daily use. It was amazing. I wondered where he got all those dogs. All us younger kids in the neighborhood looked up to James, and later I found out that he had done something quite positive with his life by joining the marines—bravely defending our country. I felt deep in my heart that he would do something great with his life.

Anyway, I didn't appreciate James's previous mockery of my mom's car, but it was a small car and James did have a dry sense of humor. That night, it was off to pick up dad in this Green Gremlin. It was July and the car's air conditioner was nonexistent. That ten-mile trip from South Side Jamaica, Queens, felt like the legendary Marathon des Sables Race through the Sahara. For those of you who do not know about this race by foot, it is a six-day marathon consisting of 156 miles of grueling, gut-wrenching, and painful trails through the Sahara with temperatures reaching 117 degrees Fahrenheit and at night 32 degrees Fahrenheit. This marathon came about from a French concert promoter named Patrick Bauer who raced 214 miles across the Sahara... BY FOOT. He went 12 days without coming across a single oasis. One thing to be careful about with ultra-marathons is hyponatremia, which is when the runner drinks too much water and dilutes the body's sodium. This electrolyte disequilibrium can be seen up to 24 hours after exercise has been completed. This dangerous decrease of sodium in the blood adversely affects the brain's operations. The decrease in sodium levels can occur due to deficits in the renal and neurohormonal systems or due to sodium loss by profuse sweating and while simultaneously taking in several pints of water. When the sodium levels outside of the cells decrease, water moves into the cells. The cells then begin to increase in size. Swelling is seen in the hands, feet, and legs. Sodium is CRITICAL in regulating the amount of water that passes through the blood– brain barrier. The decreased sodium blood levels result in increased permeability of water across the blood brain barrier. The increased entry of water causes brain swelling, which leads to shock, coma, and then death. Early symptoms that must be cautiously addressed as soon as possible are nausea, vomiting, bloating, headache, and weight gain. Pulmonary edema (water in your lungs) is also seen. Hyponatremia is a blood level where the serum sodium is less than 135 mmol/L. What is the treatment, you might ask, for hyponatremia? I would suggest fluid restriction and 100 ml of 3 percent saline hourly. Hypertonic saline is generally discontinued when neurologic symptoms have resolved, which generally occurs when the serum sodium has risen three to seven points above the initial value where symptoms have occurred. By 2009, over 1,000 runners had completed the race. Now, proceeds of the race that takes place in Morocco go to benefit health and education for the people of Morocco.

The most I ever ran was 20 miles straight, but when I hit mile ten, the runner's high kicked in and I felt invincible! I did this feat many years later in the mountains of Appalachia in West Virginia on a cool September Saturday morning. I had my Nike Air Max, and that giant callous on my left big toe was nearly unnoticeable. Thank God for a comfortable sneaker. My Air Max would usually last a year and a half and would retain its air well in the hind foot area.

Anyway, that ride in the Green Gremlin was torture. It was at least 95 degrees in the car, and that was not even counting the 100 percent humidity. I felt like a well-oiled turkey in that vehicle, minus the stuffing. We trekked onto the Interior Parkway, and to our luck, it was jam-packed with traffic. The line extended as far as the human eye could see. It was the hourglass effect: a three-lane highway now becoming a two-lane passage. I could feel my hand slowly forming a fist. I hit it hard on the side of this Green Gremlin—sorry, I mean The Emerald Green Monster—and my mother looked at me in the rearview mirror and shouted, "Boy, wait till we get home!"

Dammit. I knew one-and-a-half weeks had passed without any incident causing me to get a butt whipping! As I saw it, at least I was consistent. It was Friday, and exactly two weeks since I had my last spanking. So, I was right on time. I later took my whipping like a strong young man. I didn't even cry this time. Maybe it was the callous I felt slowly growing on my backside (from all those whippings over the past six months, like barnacles slowly fastening themselves to the side of a ship). I now had an armored Kevlar behind from the continuous belting baptism by fire.

Now, as mom and I waited in that two-lane parking lot of a traffic jam on the border of Queens and Brooklyn, a sudden breeze came rushing into the car! I said out loud, "There is a God!" "Boy, don't you be calling the Lord's name in vain!" she said. "Do you want the Holy Father to strike you down?" she shouted. I thought that God was like her—always angry. I thought that she was the Almighty's personal assassin, sort of a goddess of retribution, dispatched at the blink of an eye to judge any misdeeds that I committed. I later learned that God is caring and loving. But as a Young G back in the day, I had no access to such knowledge. As the cool breeze flowed into that four-door car I felt a sense of peace that everything would be all right. The breeze blew across face from left to right and tickled the small mustache that was starting to grow on my upper lip.

And sure enough, the traffic started to loosen up and we got to my dad's job, and mom picked up dad. Dad tried to be friendly to Ma and began with "Hi, Vera, how was your day?" "What do you mean by how was my day? I gotta come up here and bail your behind out of this mess, and I had to stop doing all my home chores—to come and pick up your behind, man!" she stated. She continued, "Ain't nobody told you to be careless and buy that car in the first place!" "It is an attractive car and you know those damn thieves like thieving them pretty cars around here! What has gotten into your head, man? You make me sick!" That cool breeze was what I needed before she went into her verbal vitriol, which could last up to 30 minutes. You would want a sinkhole to swallow you five minutes into one of her biting guilt trips. Her verbal arsenal of guilt was a well-oiled machine. It could go as long as a thirty-minute infomercial minus the productive message. When she started her tirades, it was as if the sky turned gray with cumulus clouds starting to form. You had better get out of the way or get struck by the lightning of her flying fist. I felt many times like a martial arts student avoiding an angry sensei—because like Fists of Fury, she seemed to effortlessly throw zero to 60 fists in under 1.8 seconds. Even a Lamborghini Aventador needs a "FULL" 2.6 seconds to reach its goal of zero to 60. Wow!

Anyway, she continued to tell my father, "I'm tired from this heat and this drive picking you up!" "This is what you are going to do, man," she continued. "You are going to go in that kitchen and you are going to make dinner tonight!" And you know what? That's what dad did! He knew that a happy wife is a happy home! He made some delicious chicken and rice with black beans with okra. My tongue had recovered from its prior burning at Aunt Claire's house and, man, that food was good. I really didn't care who cooked it, whether mom or dad, as long as I ate some good food. That's all I cared about as a ravenously hungry twelve-year-old boy.

Anyway, I was sad that some sucker fool had my dad's classic Ford LTD. "Dad, when you gonna get it back?" "Son, I just don't know," he responded in a dejected tone. Dad had already put in a police report there in Brooklyn at the 81st Precinct. I said, "dad, the cops got to get it fast! Don't they realize how important our family car is?" "Please, that ain't no family car—that crap's a babe magnet," my mother angrily retorted. "And I sure as hell better never see you returning any of those girls' stares either," she went on. "I see how them girls be looking at that car with you in it!" she continued. "Dear, I never see no girls looking at me in that family car," my dad responded. I loved how Pops played it off. In my dad's "innocent" eyes, that so-called babe magnet was nothing but a "family" car. But even the teenage guys would tell me that my dad's car was crazy cool and ask me if they could borrow it. To which I said, "Of course not!" In my twelve-year-old mind no amount of being cool with the older guys was worth the spanking of a lifetime. No thank you. Those callouses that I developed on my left and right backside cheeks were becoming thinner by the day as I had not been spanked for over a month. I must have been real good as the every-two-week whipping was skipped, and I didn't need the callouses reintroduced to their usual locations.

I remember why I didn't get a recent whipping. It was because I knew mom's weakness. I got her dark chocolate pecans. My butt literally was released from the leather belts of fiery justice and was on parole. When your gluteus maximus is on parole and free from being torn up by those leather belts for an extended time, it is such a relief. You feel that you are exhaling for the first time. Ahhhh.

We finally got a call from the 81st Precinct, which had located dad's babe magnet—I'm sorry, "family" car. Officer O'Leary said, "I'd like to speak with Mr. Clarence!" My dad responded, "Hello. This is he!" The officer went on, "Were you the guy that reported a stolen Ford LTD one month ago?" Dad replied, "YES!" You could really hear the childlike anticipation in his voice. It was as if he was going to get his favorite LEGO block set for Christmas. "Well," Officer O'Leary said, "we have your car. We busted a guy who was using it to commit home burglaries." My dad could hardly contain himself as he jumped up and down in excitement. His four-wheel secret love, or not so secret, depending on my mom's interpretation of things, had finally been found. My father grinned from ear to ear so widely it seemed that the rest of his face disappeared. My mother sure didn't miss a beat! She started with, "Yo, sucker, you don't smile like that for me when it’s my birthday or when our anniversary be comin’ around! How did that four-wheel Jezebel on rubber tires outrank me???” My mother was turning red in the face, and I could see that she really felt ignored. I did feel bad for her even though she tore my bottom quarters up more times than I care to remember.

So, I finally got dad all alone and asked him why Susan was acting different. She even looked different! She was at least 40 pounds lighter! Her face wore a ghoulish expression. It was as if someone or something had sucked the fat out of her face first, then the rest of her body. It was at that time beyond my childlike comprehension what was occurring inside Susan’s body that was making her drop weight like a marathoner drops sweat in a November NYC Marathon event. I simply wasn’t connecting all the dots at the ripe old age of 12. I began, “dad, she used to have a good appetite and would be more outgoing with us as a family! Now when we go by Aunt

Claire’s, she hardly comes out of her bedroom to speak with any of us.” My dad said, “She has a problem and—” “What kind of problem, dad? What type?” I thought that it was a major one for it to show such drastic changes in her so suddenly. The Susan I knew was vibrant and joyous at Christmas and Thanksgiving parties and had a bright grin with warmth that would fill the room, flowing to every corner in that room. But this Susan was now short tempered, there was no smile to be seen for miles, and this was not the cousin I knew. I felt I was beholding a clone of Susan, albeit one 40 pounds lighter with unkempt hair. So I continued to ask my dad, “Pops, I need you to explain what is really going on!” Dad gently stated, “She’s a drug addict!” I nearly turned pale and almost fell down on the carpet. Then I said, “For how long? Who is the supplier? How long will she stay in this condition? Why can’t she just stop?” Dad responded, “I know, son, it’s a lotto take in for a young boy your age.” I wanted to do so much more for my beloved cousin Susan, but there I was, totally lost in the dimension of powerlessness. It was the fourth quarter and literally the last five minutes of the game—except it was not a game. It was dead reality! I was sitting on the bench of life as it related to my cousin Susan, and the coach of intervention would not let me get a single second of playing time. Tears welled up in my eyes and stung like smoke from a burning building. I felt so much guilt as I believed I did not do enough for Susan through the years! I wanted to somehow shackle her wrist to my wrist so she could not do any self-harm, but she was older than me and I simply could not effectively restrain her. However, I vowed I would do all in my power to keep as many men, women, and children away from this monster's deadly grip.

The Pink Crystal took no prisoners. The Pink Crystal would snuff your breath out in a second, killing you with a heart attack, stroke, or respiratory arrest. This bastard just did not care. It was seductive in appearance and looked on its seductive exterior like an opulently lavish and impressive crystal that was harmless to the touch, but on the inside, it was a flaming bottomless abyss filled with burning sulfur and misery that would vaporize your mind, body, and spirit! When the addict suffers, their entire family also suffers with them! Aunt Claire would cry many times when my dad, mom, and I were over at her house having dinner. I initially wondered why, but my dad would calmly explain that Susan was doing something that she should not be doing, and on top of that, she was stealing from Auntie to get her fix. Aunt Claire would cry herself to bed many nights.

There was so much I would learn about addiction in the years to come that I had no clue about as a naive twelve-year-old. Susan's drug of choice was crack, which she smoked. It had a Pink Crystal appearance and it gave her learned as a medical student and then a physician, the paper is taken up into the lungs and then goes into the bloodstream. Once in the body, crack acts on that part of the human brain called the ventral tegmental area (VTA), and a chemical in the brain called dopamine, a neurotransmitter, is released that produces a feel-good feeling. This neurotransmitter is usually reabsorbed, but crack interrupts this cycle by binding the dopamine transporter, blocking the natural reabsorption of dopamine and producing a prolonged euphoria. Purer forms of crack rocks will sink in water or melt at the edges when near a flame and act as a local anesthetic, numbing the tongue on direct contact. The smoked formulation can create a high within ten to 15 seconds versus the snorted form, which produces a high in ten to 15 minutes.

When young people or individuals at any age get their very first high from crack cocaine, the dopamine levels in the brain are at an all-time maximum high. Later, the brain gets used to these elevated dopamine levels, and more and more of the drug is needed to achieve the same effect. However, the first high can never be reached again. This is now termed tolerance. The brain forms synaptic connections in the limbic system, aimed at getting the individual to do whatever it takes to obtain this drug. Do you remember me previously stating that there are one quadrillion synapses in the human brain with over one hundred billion nerve cells to apply all those connections? If so, it is not hard to see that the addicted individual can become extraordinarily creative in order to support his or her crack cocaine habit.

At the time, I responded to dad saying, "But, Pops, she is such a good girl. Why?" The confused look and shock on my face spoke volumes to my dad, who responded, "Drug addiction affects everyone." He said, "It does not discriminate and can affect anyone at anytime." Crack can cause heart attacks, lung hemorrhages, lack of blow flow to the bowels, stomach ulcerations for those that snort it, and intranasal ulcerations with subsequent perforation. In pregnant women, there is the problem of low birth weight, that is, less than 5.5 pounds and preterm labor before 37 weeks. Cocaine can induce urinary tract deficits, heart defects, stroke, irreversible brain damage, and even heart attacks.

Cocaine originally comes from the coca plant of the Andes Highlands of South America. The natives of this region chew or brew coca leaves into a tea to fight fatigue. Pure cocaine was first isolated in the 1880s and used as an anesthetic for eye surgery. Nose and throat surgeons in the 1800s found it particularly useful as it provided both an anesthesia and it constricted blood vessels, thereby limiting blood loss. It was even the main ingredient for Coca-Cola around 120 years ago. Crack has three phases according to "Crack Overdose: How Much Amount of Crack to OD?": 1) early stimulatory stage; 2) hyperstimulatory phase, with cardiac arrhythmias, possibly causing heart attacks and seizures; 3) depression of the central nervous system. Doses greater than five grams can induce heart attacks. Up to 75 percent of overdose deaths occur within five hours after taking crack. In 2001, crack stats showed 2 percent of college students and 4.7 percent of adults aged 19–28 used crack once in their life. About 0.9 percent and 1.3 percent used crack within the past year. Around 0.1 percent of college students and 0.4 percent of nineteen- to twenty-eight-year-olds used it in the past month, and 6.2 million Americans over the age of 12 years old tried crack once in the past year. Around one million Americans tried crack in the previous year, and another 406,000 people used crack within the past month.

At the addiction center I currently work at as the medical director, there are patients that still have cravings even six months into our program. The most difficult barrier for them when I ask them why is that even though the people they surround themselves with know that they are in a program—they don't care! A lot of my clients are so addicted to cocaine that they still use it, and I have to caution them as they are on medications that I have prescribed for their addiction.

They even tell me what I prescribe is the best thing that they have ever experienced—but it is not until they change their environment that we will both see a total change in their behavior. Some clients of mine have to literally get a U-Haul truck and move from Welch, West Virginia, and relocate up to Beckley, West Virginia. A lot of my patients have parties, and that is when they get into trouble. Some of the negative people that come to their parties bring The Other Pink Crystal Monster—crystal meth—in addition to crack, heroin, and Oxycontin. I asked one of my patients, Ms. Geeta, why her urine screen was coming back positive for Oxycontin, cocaine, crystal meth, and marijuana. This testing was also confirmed on testing several days later. I sign off on all the labs as the medical director and carefully monitor for any discrepancies. As a physician, you have to be careful about a lot of false positives. For example, Wellbutrin can cause a false positive result for methamphetamine. Moreover, Metformin (used in patients with diabetes) can cause false positivity for amphetamine and methamphetamine. Prozac and Trazadone can cause a false positive for amphetamine and methamphetamine. Sedatives for allergies can also cause false positivity for amphetamine and methamphetamine. In patients that have hypertension and are on Labetalol, they too can have false positivity for amphetamine and methamphetamine. This is the reason that, as a clinician, one must constantly be on one's toes as to other current medical comorbidities a patient has.

Anyway, Ms. Geeta responded to me, "Doc, I sort of

messed up. My hubby has been released from jail and I just had to celebrate!" I said, "And isn't there a more positive way to celebrate?" There was a long silence and, slowly looking up at me, she began, "Doc, I promise it won't happen again." As tears rolled down her face, I handed her a Kleenex. I felt for her and knew that addiction can be an uphill challenge, especially with all the brain's biochemical neurotransmitters that are involved. In fact, relapses are part of the process, and we doctors try tobrainstorm more effective ways to overcome those drug cravings. That is why, in counseling sessions, counselors try to identify triggers in the environment and how best to form an effective campaign for resistance. Ms. Geeta had been in the out-treatment center for quite a while and knew all our rules and policies. I gave Ms. Geeta credit in my subsequent encounters with her at the clinic in that she was clean for illicit drug substances. She enjoyed the counselors at our center, so that aspect of her treatment was running smoothly.

While on crack, Susan had become more promiscuous and had given birth to several children, but her mom had to be the legal guardian for the children. I want to mention that later in the same year, she had passed away because of an overdose of a pure form of crack. Susan first developed a tolerance. She required greater and greater amounts of crack to get the same effect. Crack is a stimulant, which explains why you can take it and require more and more of it, and the stimulant component of it can cause you to have a sudden heart attack. It increases the pressure within the coronary arteries and causes the blood vessel walls to rub violently against each other, resulting in stroke, heart attack, and elevated body temperature known as hyperthermia. Crack induces its "high" by enhancing the effects of the brain neurotransmitters, dopamine, serotonin, and norepinephrine, by blocking these presynaptic reuptake pumps that would normally decrease the dopamine. This causes powerful psychological effects, and people can become addicted on their very first encounter with this seductive pink and low-down dirty crystal! This form of crack has a pink crystalline appearance. My cousin Susan fought this addiction like a knight as best as she could, but in the end, it proved to be too tough a battle for her.

Now, let me revisit what causes one to become addicted to a particular drug. New synaptic connections are formed, pairing a categorical behavior with a specific reward. Now your next question might be, "How many synaptic connections exist in human beings?" That is an excellent question. Most neuroscientists believe that the average human brain contains something on the order of one quadrillion synaptic connections! How much is that equal to? Well, if I had one quadrillion dollars hanging out conveniently in my back pocket, I could give every man, woman, and child $70,000 each for just smiling at me! You sure better be giving me a good smile for me to give you my hard-earned $70,000 dollars like that in one shot! Or put another way, our very own Milky Way galaxy has around one hundred billion stars. If I were to talk about the total human synapses in the human brain, then I would need ten thousand galaxies, with each galaxy having one hundred billion stars to come close to the total number of brain connections between your two ears. Amazing, isn't it? I certainly think so. Increasing the amount of dopamine in our diet can help with some of these cravings. Foods rich in dopamine includes eggs, dairy, beets, watermelon, oatmeal, green leafy vegetables, apples, avocados, legumes, and nuts. These foods contain tyrosine, which the human body converts to dopamine. Exercise increases dopamine as well.

Back at Columbia University, alongside Professor McDermott, PhD, I had studied the distributions of these different types of receptors in the mammalian nervous system. Sociodemographic factors include early child abuse and other untreated trauma factors in 60 percent of cases of crack cocaine use. People do not turn to drugs because they are fundamentally “weak” or socially “irresponsible.” According to the National Advocates for Pregnant Women, a majority of expectant moms addicted to crack were victims of domestic violence. In my addiction medicine practice, a lot of users of drugs do so to cover up the pain from sexual abuse that started from a very early age, which is truly heartbreaking. A lot of my clients reveal to me that they simply hung out with the wrong crowd and that there was no one else for them to talk to. Others in my addiction clinic were sexually victimized and, to cope with the severe pain, turned to the other seducing Pink Crystal—crystal methamphetamine. They became so tired of being depressed that they needed a potent stimulant exactly like crystal methamphetamine that met them in the low place of despair when they were very depressed and nearly suicidal, to lift them up to heights where they could look down from the abyss of Hell that sexual abuse puts its victim into. The crystal meth had a pink glimmer crystalline appearance to it but was actually a rock from the slimy, esoteric, and formless hand of the Devil himself!

Chapter Two

Shots Fired

I took off my shoes and socks and planned out in my head as I plopped down on my bed that I was going to sleep soundly in my bed as it was 32 degrees outside in the rolling mountains of Appalachia. The sun had just set for the evening, staining the sky like a magnificent canvas overflowing and gushing with golden hues of magenta, pink, tea rose, atomic tangerine, and other splendid colors that are beyond my comprehension. According to *National Geographic*, we tend to see bright sunsets in the fall and winter in the East because the air along the path of the ray of sunlight tends to be drier and cleaner. Ice crystals slowly formed outside my window, and I thought to myself, I'm going to sleep well tonight. The ice crystals mysteriously even began to form the letter "S"—for sleep! I took it that this was a sign from the heavens that I was about to have a quiet and undisturbed sleep! I had the Honeywell thermostat locked at 78 golden degrees and had some water on the stove gently heating so that I could make the family some cocoa and discuss the events of the day.

Anyway, the colder it is outside, the deeper I sleep under that warm king-size blue and white striped comforter. It had been a busy week, and now it was 10 p.m. and I was navigating the 100 percent cotton navy-blue comforter over my face in the bed. I shift my comforter left and right for about 45 minutes every night just before falling asleep to get the perfect fit around my head. If my navy-blue comforter is not strategically positioned over my face just right, I just cannot fall asleep! It is like sleeping in the wintertime without those nice 100 percent cotton socks hugging your feet and the warmth along with it. My wife will sometimes do that thing with her ice-cold feet—touch the back of my calves and then hear me shout, “Owwweeee!” She will then calmly ask, “Babe, what’s going on?” To which I will respond, “I’ll tell you what’s going on. You just placed your ice-cold feet on my calves and now I can’t sleep!” She then looks at me with the most clueless facial expression and mutters a half-asleep “Oh, OK.” Except that it is not OK, as once I’m up it is so hard for my eyelids to become steel anchors again, plunging my body, soul, and spirit into the maritime trenches of deep and restorative sleep.

I first tried to bring the comforter slightly to the left of my face over my left eye, leaving my right eye uncovered with an opening for my mouth and nose to breathe, but that simply did not work. I then tried to bring the comforter to the right of my face over my right eye, leaving my left eye uncovered with an opening for my mouth and nose to breathe. I didn’t want even an inch of this sacred navy-blue jewel to touch the floor of our bedroom. The last time I checked under our bed, it looked like a Minnesota snowstorm in mid-January. There was white stuff delicately sprinkled on the floor alongside a hodgepodge of #2 pencils and pens. We had so many supplies under that six-foot-by-five-foot bed we could actually host a back-to-school event from all the "treasures" found there. We could actually give Walmart a run for their money! All I had to do was gift wrap those writing instruments and put a six-inch tree under our bed, and it would be Christmas 365 days a year!

Anyway, I thought that did it, as I felt myself about to descend into the world of restfulness. Then all of a sudden my wife said, "Aw, cute little baby with his comforter snuggly wrapped around his face!" I responded, "Yes, and that baby could actually sleep if you could just stop talking for five minutes, dear!" To which she responded, "Aw, the big baby is feeling kind of shy!" I countered, "No, the baby is not shy and is actually VERY tired as it has been kind of a long week." She responded, "I don't see what you are so tired from, baby. I hardly see you doing anything around here!" I replied, "Well, honey, that is why it is called work and this is called home, I see patients at work, not here in our home." She pondered these words pretty carefully and muttered a reticent, "I see." To which I responded, "Thank you. Now If you don't mind, I'm going to finally sleep." She was muttering some more words, but the sound waves were blocked out by the majestic rolling mountains of 100 percent cotton that this wondrous comforter is made up of. Her words came against the outer layer of my comforter like enemy missile fire, but my comforter did its job and strategically used its intermingling cotton inner matrix to shield my ears from her incoming, almost imperceptible, nagging explosions. Her words fell instead into the ocean of my sleep that my armored navy-blue comforter provided.

There are actually nations today, like Switzerland, that use mountains in their strategic defense against enemy invaders. Switzerland adopted a plan in the nineteenth century that basically wired entire mountains, roads, and bridges to blow up so the enemy invader would lose time trying to find inroads into the country. This was especially the case post-World War II when invasion from the Soviet Union was a very real possibility. In addition, there are many tunnels built inside the mountains that can host the entire Swiss army. Even though the Swiss have around 200,000 active military personnel, some four million citizens are actively ready for military service, too.

Anyway, there was a breach in the defenses of the navy-blue comforter's armament. It might triumphantly defend against sound from the voice missiles of peskiness, BUT it does not defend against manual tactile pressure. I promise you that I will find a solution to that one in the not-too-distant future. This very nice lady, aka the wife, took her hand and manhandled, or should I say woman handled, the comforter off my head and body and told to go to the kitchen as 1) I was supposed to make the hot cocoa and 2) the kids had a request. I responded, "Yes, dear." Upon entering the kitchen, I was greeted with, "dad, please make me some chicken!" Specifically, it was my son that was asking me to make my world-class Jamaican jerked chicken. I could hear my son's belly talking to me in rumbling torrents. He had taken his shirt off as he felt cozy with the thermostat at 78 degrees, and to my surprise, I saw the most amazing thing! Whenever his belly was rumbling from his hunger pains, I could see the skin over his entire lower belly vibrate! It appeared like a rockslide about to launch its fury on the unsuspecting motorists below. When his belly talked like this, it could surely only mean one thing, F.I.E.N.D., Food Is Emergently

Needed dad! My son can be a complete gentleman, but when the food is not ready in time, things turn into an interrogation bytes young man, like the police interrogation units would envy. He'll usually begin with "What's for dinner?" After this, the investigator—sorry, I mean son—gets past this first round of questioning, the second, tenth, and twelfth rounds of questioning are sure to follow both fast and fiendishly. The second line of questions from the investigator-son will be something along the lines of "How long does it usually take?" Before I can answer, he usually will try to answer for me. "Is it going to be five minutes, dad?" I respond, "I think a little bit longer than that, son." "Well, is it going to be ten minutes then?" "Not exactly, " I respond. "Ah, dad, please tell me that it's going to be 20 minutes!" "I'm afraid not, son," I continue to reply. He goes on, "Aw, dad, this is pure torture. Can't you speed it up?" "Sorry, son, "I'm afraid I just can't do that!" I respond. Twenty minutes, my son thinks. It takes me at least 30 minutes to prepare it the right way. In some cases, it takes me two hours to season the Jamaican chicken completely. My thoughts on chicken preparation were interrupted by a constant "BUT, BUT..." So, I said to my son, "Why are you continuing to say BUT?" "I didn't say anything," he responded. That is impossible, I think, as he is the only one here still awake. I walk from the kitchen into the living room where he is sitting on the couch and I hear the "BUT, BUT" sound. His lips are not moving at all and now I am thinking that I have a child prodigy in the art of ventriloquism in my midst! I am sure he can do this for a traveling circus and make some cash to purchase the next set of Nike's Jordans for his fast-changing foot size.

Nevertheless, that price certainly pales in comparison to the "Flu Game" of NBA legend Michael Jordan. It was Game Five of the 1997 NBA Finals, and the series was tied 2–2 with the Utah Jazz winning the last two games.

During this critical time, Jordan had the flu. No one would have blamed "His Airness" if he wanted to stay home and call out on this game, but that is simply what champions DO NOT DO! Instead, he dug deep. Deeper than an oil company drilling in the Pacific Basin way down under those billions upon billions of gallons of oceanic sea water, and he exploded in intensity as only Michael Jordan could! The Utah Jazz was leading all night long until Jordan came in like an F-5 Tornado and sequestered 15 points! Jordan gave the Bulls that much-needed win! That is why those autographed Air Jordans cost a slam-dunking, wallet-busting $105,000! He is considered by many basketball legends and historians to be the best ever to play the game. During his basketball career, Michael scored 32,292 points, earned six NBA championships, and five NBA MVP titles, and made 14 All Star appearances. He also had several Olympic gold medals on top of all these achievements.

However, it was not always like that. It was the year 1978, and Jordan was an average kid among 50 kids trying out for the Emsley A. Laney High School Varsity basketball team. The catch was that there were only 15 spots! Jordan was "only" five feet ten inches tall and at that time could not slam-dunk a basketball. The team needed a player with a good height, something that Jordan's close friend Leroy Smith had. Standing at six foot seven, Leroy was offered a spot on the team while, unbelievably, Jordan was rejected! Jordan felt humiliated and wished the ground would swallow him! He later went home that day, locked himself in a cold, isolated room, and wept inconsolably! After that, he developed a sickening maniacal basketball work ethic, and whenever he became tired from hours of endless practice, he would close his eyes and see that list in the basketball locker room without his name on it, and that catapulted him into even more intense workouts for several more hours. The rest is NBA history!

Anyway, I heard it again—"BUT, BUT, BUT"—and, much to my amazement, his lips were not moving an inch! Well, I was thinking to myself, I have not eaten all day but I am not delirious. I walked up closer to where I could hear "BUT, BUT, BUT." I traced the mysterious sound until I came closer to its origin! Sure enough, I heard the sound again and my ear lit onto a mountainous domain where this sound was coming from. I diligently looked at our smoke detectors. Nope, that was not where it was coming from. Then I proceeded to check the phones as all sorts of sounds come from them! No, it was not the phones either! Well, where in the world could it be coming from? "BUT, BUT, BUT." It began again. I asked my son once more, "Young Man, where is that sound coming from?" "Dad, you know that I don't know!" I knew he was getting testy as his hunger pains can get the best of him and an attitude is sure to ensue. I moved by instinct to the sound of "BUT, BUT, BUT" where my ear lit on the mountainous shape of my son's belly! The sound of his hunger pains sounded just like "BUT, BUT, BUT!" I revealed my discovery to him. "Son, your belly, whenever you are hungry, it makes the sound of a deep 'BUT, BUT, BUT.'" I give that response to the wife when I promise her the alarms will not go off the next time I cook!

Anyway, to make this sumptuous treat, I added salt, black pepper, sage, special jerk chicken powder, leeks, onions, and shredded carrots to a bed of olive oil sitting on top of some Reynolds wrap in a twelve-inch-by-eighteen-inch iron pan. I placed around 12–14 pieces of chicken in there and set the oven at 425 degrees for one hour and 45 minutes.

Let me tell you about the benefits of these ingredients that I use. Sage can reverse the signs of aging—wrinkles, age spots, fine lines. Sage is also rich in calcium and vitamin A. Sage protects against free radicals and delays the onset of facial wrinkles. It has anti-inflammatory properties and antiseptic properties too. Those of us that suffer from eczema and psoriasis can use it. Sage also stimulates hair growth. It has beta-sitosterol, which has been proven to be effective in combating male pattern baldness. A combination of rosemary and sage will make hair thicker, darker, and shinier. A sage and rosemary rinse is created by boiling the two herbs in water. Did you also know that sage is used to treat sore throats and inflamed tonsils? For this, you boil some sage leaves in about 12 ounces of water. Add some honey to it, and when the sage brew comes back down to room temperature, you can use it to gargle every eight hours for sore throat relief. Do you have problems with indigestion? Well, sage can help with bile flow, intestinal mobility, and relieve an upset stomach. Do you have upper airway problems? Sage when mixed with water can be placed in a humidifier and acts as a natural smooth muscle relaxant, thereby relaxing the smooth muscles of the airway to help during an asthma attack. It also helps in removing mucous congestion in the airways. Do you have problems with diabetes? Sage has blood sugar-lowering properties. By blocking the release of stored glucose from the liver, it can help reduce your sugar levels tremendously. Do you have a loved one with Alzheimer's? The regular intake of sage has been found to increase acetylcholinesterase levels in the human brain. Acetylcholinesterase improves concentration and treats memory loss seen in Alzheimer's. Feeling sad and just cannot get over it? Well, sage tea can help you deal with depression and grief. How many ladies out there are suffering from hot flashes? No, I am definitely not calling you beautiful mature ladies old! Definitely not! We as younger people can learn from those that are mature in years, chronologically speaking. Well, sage is great for some of the menopausal symptoms of hot flashes and excessive sweating. Used as a dry leaf extract, it can reduce sweating by 50 percent. Are you just overwhelmed by the thought of a noxious boss come Monday morning? Sage has other properties that, when it is used in aromatherapy, alleviate nervousness, fatigue, tiredness, anxiety, and headaches. Combat those Monday morning blues with confidence! Sage is also a natural meat preserver. It can add a little extra shelf life if you season your meats with this very valuable spice.

Next, let us talk about leeks, which I use while cooking my chicken. We see in the Old Testament, in numbers 11:5, that after the ancient Israelites are free from Egypt, they complain against Moses and state, “We remember the fish, which we did eat in Egypt freely; the cucumbers, and the melons, and the leeks, and the onions and the garlic.” Boy, that one text in the Bible sure is making me hungry as I write this. We see here that they had leeks thousands of years ago. Furthermore, leeks were highly prized by the Greeks and Romans for the effects on the throat. The Greek philosopher Aristotle attributed the clear voice of a partridge to leeks, and it was thought that the Roman emperor Nero ate leeks daily to make his voice sound stronger! Leeks are related to onions, and the white base is edible, while the dark green sheaths at the top may be discarded. Please come with me as we delve into the health benefits of leeks. Leeks contain allicin, which has antibacterial, antifungal, and antiviral properties, and leeks produce a compound by the name of sulfuric acid that is evidenced to neutralize toxic-free radicals quicker than any other known compound. In addition, leeks contain an antioxidant called kaemferol, which is found in kale, broccoli, and cabbage. Kaemferol, in turn, has antimicrobial, anti-inflammatory, cardioprotective, and antidiabetic properties. It also has analgesic, anti-allergy, and anxiety-reducing properties. Since leeks are related to chives, shallots, onions, and garlic, the types of cancer that leeks can help protect against include prostate, colon, and stomach cancer. Folate is rich in 5-methyltetrahydrofolate [5-MHTF], which is a cardioprotective compound.

Let us look at some other benefits that leeks have to offer. Leeks are a good source of prebiotics. Many of us already know about probiotics. However, do you know the difference between a prebiotic and a probiotic? Let me explain. Probiotics are live bacteria found in yogurt and other dairy products. Probiotics are frequently prescribed by a physician to prevent severe diarrhea, bloating, and cramping as side effects from taking a prescribed antibiotic for any number of medical reasons. However, probiotics can be destroyed by heat and stomach acid, defeating the purpose they were intended for even before they have a chance to act. We also do not know which good bacteria our individual bowels require as everyone's body functions in a different manner.

Now let me explain a prebiotic to you. It is a plant fiber that nourishes and promotes the “good” bacteria already present in your bowel! A prebiotic is a fertilizer allowing the “good” bacteria that are already there to thrive! A prebiotic optimizes the ratio of good to bad bacteria. Patients who consume probiotics daily have fewer problems with depression and anxiety. Probiotics are not affected by heat or acid.

Let us move on to onions. Loaded with vitamin C, they boost your immunity, and vitamin C helps with the absorption of iron, thereby aiding those of us that suffer from anemia. If you feel tired all the time, you may not be taking in enough vitamin C in your diet. Of course, you can consume more oranges, which may be more palatable than consuming three or four raw onions! Onions contain chromium, which regulates blood sugar. Onions also lower LDL, the bad cholesterol. Onions have a powerful compound that is cancer fighting as well, and it is called quercetin. Onion juice is also an instant remedy for bee stings. Shallots and Western yellow onions are the healthiest. Do you suffer from insomnia? Onion soup can help you get the sleep you rightfully deserve without having to worry about the unnecessary side effects of a sleeping pill, some that may cause respiratory depression. Onions also are loaded with manganese, which is useful in the defense against the common cold and flu.

Now when it comes to cooking, I tend to cook at one o'clock in the afternoon. Cooking puts me in another dimension of "relaxation" and allows me to unwind after a stressful day of work. So, when my son asked me to make some Jamaican chicken, it was a relaxing way for me to end my evening! My son began, "dad, that chicken sure smells good!" I responded, "Son, it's going to be at least another hour. I just put it in the oven!" To which he responded, “Aw, man, it smells so good. Can we do it any faster?” “I’m afraid not, son,” I replied. My son went on, “Well, why not?” I responded, “Son, you just can’t. When you cook for your family later on, you too will see why!” I was thinking to myself, does this boy want a raw bird inside of him?

We were just coming from basketball practice and his Nike basketball sneakers had been giving us a run for our money in every possible way. I sprayed some Febreze Linen & Sky Air freshener in the shoes. So that my wife would not pass out. The odor of those sneakers was canceling out the wondrous aroma of my Jamaican chicken! Anyway, this boy’s feet can grow. I have to purchase new sneakers as frequently as we purchase eight-ounce Styrofoam cups from Walmart! Instead of the speed of light being the fastest unit of velocity in the universe, it should be the speed of the increase of foot size in a nine-year-old boy. This new unit of speed, I assure you, is the fastest metric I can think of! Just ask any parent with a young sprouting one about the effects it has on their wallet! Those 50 dollars you thought you were going to spend on changing your vehicle's oil has now evaporated on yet another set of new sneakers. Moreover, they want the Jordans, or shoe brands endorsed by other famous athletes! To me, it seems that every athlete now has a sneaker. They also come in a range of colors. There is magenta, periwinkle, salmon, amaranth purple, quinacridone magenta, and navy-blue colored basketball sneakers.

My son started to play the drums, hitting a slew of sixteenth notes on the snare drums and tom-tom. I love music a lot, but at this hour? Well, it is a labor of love. As long as he learns to play an instrument, I guess it is alright. I had taken my earplugs and had prepared to sit down to read my Bible for the evening when, all of a sudden, I heard a thunderous shriek. "Daaaaaaad, come here!" my daughter suddenly screamed. I dropped my Bible on the bed and ran in her direction. She ran out of her bedroom at the same time and we almost had a collision! "What's the matter, dear?" She was nearly turning pale and just pointed to the east side of her room. I responded, "Baby, if dad is to help you, you've got to tell me what's going on!" Her little lips were just quivering and I saw a little tear well up in the corner of her left eye. She grabbed me by the right shoulder and with all her might mustered enough energy from her little diaphragm to say, "Look over there!" My wife was asleep at this time and when she heard our daughter scream, she said, "Isaac, is everything alright? Are you burning the house down?" I responded indignantly, "Babe, what is it with you? Why is it that every time I cook, you mention that something is burning?" My wife without missing a beat responded, "Babe, last time you were cooking, don't you remember the fire alarms going off at like 100 decibels, and we thought the Fire Department was about to come?" I played it off as I did not want to inflate my wife's planetary-sized ego. Her ego with regard to my cooking was so big that it had planetary moons revolving around it. The moons surrounding her planetary-sized ego related to my cooking could initiate 100-foot-high tidal waves that only a Hawaiian surfer would appreciate. I said to my dearest wife, "Honey, I have no idea what you are referring to!" She quietly gave me the stare. I responded, "What, baby?" She responded, "You know what! You, kitchens, and fire alarms just don't get along!"

Anyway, I did not pursue this topic with the "boss" of the house. As the underboss, I knew my rightful place and I raised the white flag verbally by simply responding with one of my most classic "Yes, dear's!" that was available. That instantly ended any possible issue so I could quickly go back to my daughter, who was in apparent distress. My daughter was still pointing toward the east side of her bedroom. I instantaneously gazed in the direction of her elongated index finger. I stared at the spot as hard as I could, but I still could not see anything. "Honey, I don't see a thing"—But before I could get another word out, she screamed, "Ahhhhhhhhhhhhhh! There it goes, Daddy!" "What is it?" I responded. "It's... It's..." Her lips again quivered and I just held her by both shoulders and said, "Honey, take a deep breath, in and out five times." She did this, and her pallor disappeared and the color returned to her face. She was now more calm and collected. I begin, "Dear, can you talk now?" She responded with another "Ahhhhhhhhhhhh!" I understood this was going nowhere fast, so I coincidentally looked over my left shoulder toward the east side of her room and observed a black jumping spider. I looked my daughter in the eyes and I said, "Ahhhhhhhhhhhhhhhhhhhhhhhhhhhhhhhhhhhhhhhhh!!!!!"

I am sorry. That ugly thing was looking at me with 12 eyes and I was thinking, this was not natural. At least Jesus had 12 blessed disciples helping him as his assisting eyes! This critter had 12 wretched eyes that were terrorizing my daughter and me! Quite the opposite of what our good Lord was doing! When you have as many eyes as I have toes on both feet, and then on top of that, throw in a few fingers for the final tally, you have to go! I quickly spotted an old Nike shoebox, and this large critter effortlessly jumped into the box as if he was qualifying for the gold medal at a track and field event! I closed the box and as calmly as I could, released the spider on the outside lawn far, far away from my home. I was as speechless as my daughter had been just five minutes earlier. Now, with this twelve-eyed villain out of our home, my daughter could talk again! "Dad," she began, "Are you OK? You don't look so good!" I caught my breath and followed the same advice that I had given to her earlier. I swallowed five enormous breaths, nearly forgetting to exhale, to which my daughter said very confidently, “Dad, you know you got to let those breaths out!” When I did release those breaths, I saw a thousand stars glittering in front of my eyes. My daughter continued, “You going to speak or what?” I finally pulled up a chair and saw why she was speechless. I began, “That was the ugliest and fastest-moving spider I have ever seen in my life!” That sucker raised its front legs and looked at me with those 12 despicable eyes while supporting the rest of its weight effortlessly on its hind legs. It was defying all the laws of physics that I had learned back in college, and I felt a shiver go down my spine!

Anyway, the Jamaican chicken had another 30 minutes to go, and my son began saying, “Daaaad, I’m really hungry!” I responded, “Let’s do some homework.” We mutually decided to review his math. When I looked at the first problem, it was a simple equation "1X + 2C = 5Z."

We worked at this equation together and then proceeded to do several more problems equivalent to this first equation. When I looked at the next set of equations, there were more letters in it than numbers, and it seemed like a Pac-Man game, where with the passage of time, the numbers, like the pellets, all disappear! All that is left are those darned letters with each new equation representing the blank space remaining after Pac-Man has feasted on his sumptuous pellets. I felt bad for the poor numbers as they were decreasing through no fault of their own, while those overzealous letters were multiplying like rabbits! Those poor numbers were like an endangered species, and I felt like I needed to petition Congress to create an endangered species preservation society for that ever-decreasing concentration of numbers in all those darned equations!

I looked up at the wall clock, and, sure enough, it was time to retrieve the chicken from the oven so that my fire alarms would not go off—again! If I was ever to take up the cause of those poor little numbers by helping them form their own endangered society, I would first have to do so with some food in my stomach. Having a full stomach would give me the necessary energy to fight and gain strategic ground to preserve the dignity and identity of those dwindling special numbers in my son's algebraic equations. My son looked at me with those sad puppy eyes and muttered, "Dad is it done already?" To which I responded, "Yep, it's time for some chicken indeed!" All those math equations made me so hungry that I raced to the kitchen and discovered 14 golden brown chicken drumsticks looking at me. Each one of those golden brown honey-glazed Jamaican jerk chicken drumsticks had some chopped chives on top with diced carrots. My mouth was watering, and I had some green beans and brown rice to go along with this sumptuous treat. I served my son first, and then I jumped into the feast after him. I knew that both of us, my son and I, would need full stomachs to conquer that alien army of invading letters in my son's math homework.

Once I had my fill of some good food, my eyes that were once dim were now wide open and I could face a planet full of letters and not move a single muscle in fear as we both tackled those indomitable mathematical equations. My son's jaws were moving like crossheads on the wheels of a steam locomotive train. Faster and faster and yet faster it went. His jaws, powered by the master, temporal, and pterygoid muscles of the face and jaw, were reaching new heights of locomotive fury. Faster and faster they moved! At this point, I was afraid that he might bite his tongue or become the real-life CPR doll on which I would have to do the Heimlich maneuver. Nothing was slowing the circular motion of his chewing jaws, which at this point had reached an all-time frenzy. “Son, please slow down!” I shouted. The chewing continued unabated in its high-velocity endeavor. I spoke just a little bit louder, “Son, chew slower!” But there was still no response. I was thinking to myself—what would it take to get this boy’s attention? I thought I had the answer because this boy has selective hearing.

My dear fellow parents, you may know what I mean. The kind of selective hearing that can hear when you say, “Hey, everybody, I have pizza and soda!” but 10 seconds later when you say, “I want one of you kids to clean the bathroom floor, please, after you finish eating the pizza” and no one responds. Yes, I am talking about that kind of selective hearing. My son plays it off when I tell him, “Clean your room!” He usually responds, “Huh? Pick up the spoon? Dad, did you say pick up the spoon?” “No, that’s simply not what I said, son,” I tell him. Obviously, picking up a spoon is effortless and takes three seconds to do, while cleaning his bedroom, when done properly, takes up to an hour—such a clever kid!

Anyway, my words of caution went unheard and he continued to chew faster than a Milwaukee 4-4-2 locomotive train traveling 80 miles per hour! I knew how I could deal with my son's selective hearing. I walked over to the living room and held up a block set of LEGO Super Heroes. I called out, "Hello, son!," this time waving the LEGO block set where his peripheral vision was sure NOT to miss. The jaws of the locomotive frenzy slammed to a grinding halt! They did not even coast down the tracks for 10 feet. They slammed to a sudden lockdown! "Dad, I didn't know you still had the box!" he screamed with excitement. I responded, "Why, of course!" I would never dare throw that box out as any one of those 175 razor-sharp daggers would be way too eager to put their ferocious teeth into the bottom of my feet at one in the morning when I have to answer the call of nature. The boy ran at me faster than a lion about to take down a 1,000-pound wildebeest across the grasslands of southeastern Angola and Namibia. My son took another bite of the Jamaican chicken, but this time he took a huge chunk out of it, bigger than he had ever taken before.

Anyway, he was completely unaware that the box that I was currently holding, out of the 175 pieces that this LEGO block set contained, only two pieces were in the actual box! Now, I know you might be asking the question: Where are the remaining 173 pieces? Splendid question, folks! I know where they are, but my son does not. You may wonder as to how I can be so sure of this fact. Well, that is because he was still running full speed in my direction, interspersed with twisting himself in a circle—sort of running one foot, then twirling in a circle for another two feet. On and on, this goes in a rhythmic fashion. You remember what I mentioned previously about selective hearing. Well, sometimes that selective hearing is also paired with selective seeing. I put my hand out and loudly said to the young steam locomotive, “STOP NOW!” My son mysteriously saw neither my hand gesturing him to stop nor did he hear my loud declaration to stop as he ran full speed on top of 25 of those LEGO blocks, out of the 173 that were on the floor, which went into his foot! “Oww!” the young boy cried. He had been ambushed by the army of LEGO blocks that he had refused to put away for the night—for every night! Next thing I saw was the chicken fly out of his mouth, across the room, and onto my snare drum. Not good. I preferred the traditional moongel to be on my snare, hi toms, low toms, and bass toms. I certainly did not need a piece of chicken to lower the higher overtones of my percussion instruments!

“Dad, dad, you gotta help me!” Now we see where my son’s selective hearing and seeing has gotten him! I then adopt selective comprehension as the adult parent. “Dad, are you listening?" he continued. "What's the matter, son?" I responded. "Look, look—it's stuck!" My selective comprehension is like a politician—it is just starting to serve its public office but still cannot grasp the implications of its full duties! Again my son yelled, "Dad, it's stuck!" To which I responded, "What's stuck and where?" I had already surveyed the landscape beneath my feet, which were fortunate enough to be nestled intimately in the confines of my thick black and white Adidas leather slippers. My son, on the other hand, was always going barefoot. "Dad, come on now!" I decided that he had learned his lesson and proceeded to help him. They came out easily, but one had penetrated the skin and I pulled it out slowly and gently, and his foot began bleeding. "Dad, it hurts!" I tried to encourage him but to no avail. Again, he said, "Make it stop!" I expeditiously got some water and sterilely cleaned the sole of his foot, put a topical antibiotic on it, placed a fabric Band-Aid on it, and then wrapped it with gauze. After finishing dinner, my son said, "I'm too tired to do those equations!" I responded, "Sounds reasonable to me." He hobbled and limped his way to bed to sleep for the night after sustaining an assault by those lethal LEGO blocks. I would need a full belly and a full eight hours of sleep before even letting the thought enter my mind of wanting to attack that army of mathematical equations with those advancing letters that awaited us in the morning. I knew those poor little numbers in those algebraic equations were no match for those resilient letters. In one of those equations, it could be an "A" or it could be a "Z," or it could be sinister enough to be a double combination following behind a poor number, like "1BC + 4BC = 12C." Now, why in the world does that poor little number 1 have to be followed by those relentless "Bs and Cs"? I could feel a tear forming in the corner of my eye every time I saw this double assault happening on those poor little numbers!

I finally fed the rest of the family and was off to bed. I got my full eight hours of sleep and felt refreshed when I woke up the next morning. My son and I worked on his math homework with renewed vigor, and all the assaults from those letters in the algebraic equations seemed to vanish as we slayed them one by one. He brought home his math report card three weeks later and he had scored 95 marks—a straight "A"; mission accomplished! That is the only letter I like to see, and the appropriate place where I enjoy seeing it the most—on his report card. However, I did not let my guard down as I knew those letters were coming back with specialized reinforcements. When they landed with all boots on ground, I knew they were going to be in a frenzy of activity caused by a fermenting vengeance, unleashing triple-letter equations like "2DEG + 7DEG= 13G." I mean, talk about vicious! However, we will be prepared. We will get reinforcements for those poor small numbers—this time called “million, billion, and trillion!”

Anyway, as I closed my son’s math book, I put on my sneakers, went outside, and ran for three miles. Along the way, I spotted an owl looking dead at me from a mockernut hickory tree. I ran, getting closer, closer, closer to that tree, with this owl still eyeing me, and in between, blinking with these humungous eyes, he decided to rotate his head nearly 300 degrees. I was thinking this bird was possessed when, all of a sudden, this brown-colored Barred Owl swooped down to take a closer look at me! His wingspan was at least three feet across, and I had not realized how fast he could actually move. The bird must have thought I was a giant eastern chipmunk because he swooped down toward me and instantly realized I was much bigger than he could have ever imagined. He quickly rode the air current, which carried him in its air pocket to a branch 50 feet up. He looked at me with a kind of disappointed look in his eye, wishing I could have been a nice morning snack before something more substantial came along. I looked at him in stern consternation, letting him know that he would never get that close to me again. Of all the hundreds of acres of air space to fly in, he decided that he had to violate my airspace and swoop down within one foot of my face.

I instinctively ducked low to the ground and while I was in that position managed to see a hickory tussock moth caterpillar. It was mildly crossing the road and it looked so fuzzy, and I thought I would pick it up. But wait. If I recall correctly, those two long black hairs—one at the front and the other at the rear—are connected to poison glands that excrete venom on contact. The response to human skin ranges from mild hives to possibly bulla on the skin with fevers, chills, and drenching sweats. The treatment is to wash the affected area with soap and water, take an antihistamine like Benadryl, and use calamine lotion and an ice pack.

Anyway, this caterpillar just wished to be left alone, and I let it have its wish and continued my jog.

The trail I run on is full of peaks and valleys, and the callous on my left big toe was burning like an acetylene torch. The hot searing pain was intensifying as I made my way uphill. Foot after foot, I advanced slowly as I was not there to run the four-minute mile. The pain was temporarily neutralized when drops of sweat went into my eye, creating a burning sensation, and then I mysteriously could not feel the pain in my foot any longer. I took my navy-blue washcloth and wiped my brow, careful not to send any more of that sulfuric acid-type sweat into my already tenderized eyeballs.

The human eye is amazing. It can see the Andromeda galaxy some 2.5 million light years away in outer space, but if you dare to get a single eyelash in it, it is as if your whole body shuts down. The eye almost goes entirely dim. I remember when I had my LASIK eye surgery, I went from being almost near blind to having fighter pilot vision, with my left eye being 20/20 and my right eye being slightly better at 20/15. I just had to have that surgery, as I was tired of wearing my spectacles that were shaped like Coca-Cola bottom glasses and used to fall off during basketball games, being crushed by a fellow player's size 14 sneaker. I remember sometimes playing without those glasses 20 years ago and winning a vicious elbow to the groin, which resulted in me reaching a higher choral pitch than even the pastor's sister singing the morning hymn! I was also elbowed in the eye with those darned eyeglasses and nearly had my nose broken. When we played basketball, it was a conquest of manhood. We would play our basketball like football mixed with the likes of rugby minus the grass—as we played exclusively on asphalt. I twisted my ankles many times when going for rebounds, and landed on my ankle from a near three-foot vertical leap that I could do once upon a time. I later had that LASIK surgery and it was a game changer. It was as if God took some mud and water and handcrafted a new cornea and retina for me because, for the first time, I could see people that I had not been able to see without my glasses. Several hours after the surgery, it was like I could see the "trees" (referring to how people looked like blurred objects to me without my glasses) walking for the very first time. One of my friends, Patrick, remarked "Yo, Zac. I held my hand up high in the street to say, 'What's up?' and you never responded!" I replied, "That's because I never saw you!" Patrick replied, "How is that possible?" I responded, "I just can't see!" To which he responded, "I wasn't even that far away from you!" I responded, "Just exactly how far away were you?" He responded, "Twenty feet!" I then told him, "That's why!" Patrick responded, "That's why what?" To which I responded, "Man, anything greater than two feet and I can't make out your face!" To which he responded bluntly, "You as blind as the federal government seeing that it gets an income tax return to the rightful owners!" I responded, "That's cruel, man, just cruel!"

Anyway, I continued on my running trail and I saw a mockernut hickory tree's leaf make its descent through the air from the top branch, some 20 feet above me. It was twisting and then shifting to the left, so I quickly ran to the left, and it then abruptly changed its trajectory and swung to the right, falling down even faster. I made adjustments and suddenly darted to the right of the road, but it changed its trajectory again. This time it decided to fall behind me very suddenly and was about five feet above me falling fiercely. I stayed frozen in place, not looking to make another move. Then, suddenly, it was one foot over my head, and I leaped explosively in its direction, opened my hand, and grabbed it. I just enjoy catching leaves when I run.

So, I completed my run, showered, and took the family out for lunch. Later that weekend, we went to church on Sunday, and then I went to bed at 10 o'clock that night, getting ready for an unpredictable Monday morning. When I get at least eight hours of sleep, I can think on my toes.

It was now six in the morning and my alarm went off, so I walked 20 feet to the kitchen to make coffee for the wife, and made a left to get near the cupboard where I keep the coffee powder. Just as I was about to make another left, I stepped on it! "Ouch!" I cried out. That boy of mine still had not picked up the remaining LEGO blocks, and one managed to pierce my foot, causing some blood to spurt. The wife began, "Did you make my coffee?" I responded, "I will soon make it!" She responded, "Why soon and not right away?" I said, "Because our son forgot to put up his LEGOs for the night." She responded, "So, get to it!" Looking to save time and not engage the boss, being the underboss that I am, I simply responded, a half-awake and half-asleep, ”Yes, dear!” She continued, “And I don’t want it wimpy, baby. You gotta make it strong!” That sounded somewhat romantic for a second, and a sly grin raced across my face. However, I did not have time to ponder on it much as time flies on a Monday morning when you are dropping the kids off at school and then have to get to work.

I arrived at my addiction center and greeted my staff. “Hi, Ms. G.” “Hello, Dr. Alexis” she responded. I greeted the lab personnel, counselors, and the rest of my staff. I settled down in my office and logged onto my computer to see the list of patients that I would be seeing for the day. I noticed that I would be seeing several new patients, which I immensely enjoy because I want to make a difference in all my wonderful patients’ lives, those that are suffering from drug addiction.

I saw my first patient, Mr. Z. He had been fighting his addiction to crack cocaine for the past 20 years, which had resulted in him losing his marriage. He had tears in his eyes because he was about to lose his child. I said, "Mr. Z, What's going on today?" He responded, "Doc, I just don't know what to do!" I responded, "Tell me about it!" He continued, "I don't know if I'm going to see my son ever again!" My heart breaks every time I hear stories of a parent losing custody of their child. However, a child must have a stable environment to thrive spiritually, academically, and socially. About three months into my program, Mr. Z was abusing the Pink Crystal drug (crack) much less, and the courts deemed him responsible enough to have his son back. He came in one day and said, "Doc, Doc, you simply won't believe what just happened!" Iresponded, "Mr. Z, I'm excited. Tell me, tell me!" To which he responded, "Well, Doc, I got my son back!" I nearly jumped and hit the ceiling with my head (the ceilings of the center are low, only about seven and a half feet high).

When I first met Mr. Z, he was on edge. Every muscle in his body was twitching from head to toe, he was sweating profusely and would blink his eyes a thousand times a minute. He was in withdrawal as he was detoxing from crack cocaine, which he had been using for over 20 years. In our program, we started him on medicines that would ease the withdrawal symptoms while simultaneously decreasing any of his cravings for crack cocaine. At his first meeting with me, he mentioned some of the social trials and tribulations that he was going through, and my heart wept for him. I believe in the power of Jesus to break through the spiritual component of addiction in addition to the brain biochemical and brain physiological responses to addiction. So we prayed together because, as mentioned in Matthew 18:20, "where two or three are gathered together in my name, there am I in the midst of them." I sincerely believed in Mr. Z. There was that burning sensation in my soul that he really wanted to change. When I first met him, the first words that came out of his mouth were, "Doc, I'm doing this for my son." I responded, "I believe you, man." Mr. Z continued, "Doc, with all my heart, I want a better life for me and my son. I just can't go on living like this." I responded, "I'm going to do everything in my power to help you as much as possible." I held his hand and asked if he would like to pray. I never force anyone to pray, but I sincerely believe that prayer works. I started, "Dear Father God, in the blessed and infinite name of Jesus, please help Mr. Z in all that he is facing and please break the power and spirit of addiction and help Mr. Z be reunited with his family, in particular, his son, dear Lord, in the name of Jesus, the son of the Living God, and please make all crooked pathsbecome straight as he continues on the road to recovery. Amen." Mr. Z put his hat back on with tears in his eyes and said, “Thanks, Doc. That’s exactly what I needed!”

I want all my patients to be relaxed when they are at my center; relaxed in the sense that this is a judgment-free zone and no one will judge them here. However, even though I want them to feel relaxed, I want them to put their whole heart, mind, and soul into the recovery process as addiction is a serious issue. That means separating themselves from bad influences such as “old friends” and acquaintances who will thrust a dirty crack pipe every time they see my clients at a family reunion, Christmas gathering, or New Year’s celebration. I have had clients that, no matter how many times I tell them that they can test positive for crystal meth after it should have cleared out of their body looking at urine drug screens from about three to seven days. It can also take longer if the individual has been a longtime user. Many patients continue to lie to my face and tell me that they have quit using the drug when their urine is still testing positive two months later. Accountability is critical to their success. If a client is lying to me, we are on a very slippery slope, and no one benefits in that relationship. Some patients that are dead set on success rent a U-Haul truck and literally trek their life's belongings and move away from the people, sights, sounds, and smells that could and would trigger a relapse in their quest to stay "clean." They are the successful ones at my clinic. In reality, it is a function of them absolutely refusing to stop hanging with bad company. For around 90 percent of them, this means not going to the same parties where illicit substances are shared alongside food and drinks.

Mr. Z is one of our success stories in that he now rarely tests positive for crack cocaine and, I am happy to say that now he has full custody of his son. In the past, no matter how much counseling he went through, initially, he often did test positive for cocaine. When I knocked on the door of the examination room, he would begin, “Yes, Doc, I know it’s positive but all my neighbors are selling it. What do I do?” It is not as if he has a million dollars and can just move out of his current environment. That is why I encourage my patients to read newspapers and be on the lookout for any possible job openings. Reading, first, keeps the mind occupied and keeps many of my patients out of trouble. More importantly, reading increases the release of brain dopamine, which gives a sense of euphoria and decreases the desire even to abuse drugs. Anyway, he is the best that I have seen him in months, and I could not be happier for him. By the grace of God alone, and to Jesus be all the Glory!

My next patient is a new patient by the name of Ms. J. Ms. J was sexually assaulted by her father and his friends at the age of 10, and was driven to try to commit suicide because of this diabolic act perpetrated against her. She slit her wrist numerous times and showed me the healed scars across her wrist. To stop the pain, she ran away with a boyfriend 20 years her senior, and to suppress all the pain she had experienced after numerous vicious rapes by her father, could only cope to see another day when she was high on crystal methamphetamine. Ms. J was around five feet tall and 250 pounds. She had an amiable personality when she came to our center. The first words out of her mouth were, “Doctor, I have something to say!” I responded, “Please, Ms. J, tell me what’s going on.” She responded, “Well, Doctor, when I was 10 years old, I didn’t want to live anymore!” I responded, “Please tell me why.” Ms. J responded, “My dad...” Tears begin to well up in her eyes and I offered her a Kleenex. She continued talking, “He raped me at the age of 10 along with his friends and stepbrothers.” I was absolutely horrified by what I was hearing and my eyes began to burn as I was tearing up as well. She continued, “While I was out of state, my boyfriend and I were in trouble with the law and got arrested." I asked her, "What led to you getting arrested?" She replied, "Well, Doc, I had an expensive crystal methamphetamine and crack habit and I had to spend $600–$1,000 daily just to maintain my habit!" She then continued, "I did things that I was ashamed of, like stealing from other people—a lot." She continued, "We were running from the law at night and sleeping in cars in the daytime and staying in abandoned homes and homeless shelters just to survive!" I asked, "Ms. J, why specifically crack and crystal methamphetamine?" She responded, "My boyfriend introduced me to it and it was great!" She continued, "The crack and crystal meth gave me a release from the prison of shame from being raped by my father." She continued, "I felt on top of the world and I felt that I could conquer anything!" Words do not express how bad I felt for her at this moment. I wanted to have a face-to-face conversation with this animal of a human being that tried to destroy his ten-year-old daughter on multiple levels. She then hung her head low, and her brunette hair freely hung down, covering her face that had become beet red after this confession to me. I replied, "Ms. J, I am here to help you with our group of counselors and I will never judge you." She replied, "Thanks, Doc."

She then continued, "Other things happened to me too. I was kidnapped and raped while in a state of unconsciousness and the guy urinated on me!" I was absolutely appalled at what I had just heard and felt powerless as a physician. What could I do to offer this damaged soul hope of a second life? She needed a mental transformation and a new will to combat her abusive past. She continued, "And oh, by the way, I was sleeping in an apartment with my boyfriend when some gang members kicked out our windows and did the unthinkable!" I screamed in a frenzy, "Ms. J, what did they do?" Ms. J continued, “Well, after they kicked in the windows, the next thing I saw was a hand and in it was a rifle!” I was petrified hearing this and was inwardly praying that no one was killed during the night. Ms. J continued, ”They pulled the trigger and start releasing round after round of gunfire, and I jumped out of that room as I felt one of the bullets whiz right past my left temple!”

I was completely shocked by the beyond comprehensible trauma that this young lady had had to endure! I then asked, “Ms. J, what did you do next?” to which she responded, “I saw sparks of fire coming out of that rifle, and all I could think to do was duck down—and fast!” I responded, “Then what happened?” Ms. J said, “The bastard continued to shoot rounds at the door, so that I couldn’t escape, blocking my exit!” She continued, “I looked up to the heavens, praying to God that I survive because I thought I might not.” She continued, “So he put one foot through the window, and he was wearing this white and maroon baseball cap with sunglasses; I couldn't even make eye contact with the dude!" Ms. J went on, "If he had his glasses off, I could at least see what his intentions were, but he wore a stone-cold expression!" She felt totally trapped at this point, as the murderer did not telegraph what he was going to do next. She went on to describe the perpetrator. "This guy then put his right hand on the ledge of the window, and he had the biggest hands I'd ever seen in my life. He was wearing black leather gloves, I guess to conceal his fingerprints so there wouldn't be any physical evidence from whatever he left behind. He then violently pushed at the wall at least seven times. I was totally freaking out and could not even imagine what this guy was about to do next! I felt as if the brown painted room was getting smaller and smaller every time I blinked my eyes! Every second felt like an hour, and I couldn't wait to get the heck out of there. Sweat was pouring down both sides of my face, and I tried to prevent it from going in my eyes because given how dangerous this dude was, if I lost my line of sight for one second, I knew he could hurt me—hurt me a lot!

Ticktock. Another second passed; the room was growing ever smaller, and I felt as if I was in a closed coffin, as I couldn't even get my chest to take in some air, let alone release it! He again pulled off some more shots, and one of the bullets hit the mattress, went right through it, and tore right into both of my shoes, so now I had nothing to run away from him. He pulled off four more shots. One went into a giant glass vase we had, shattering it into a million pieces and sending all the fragments exploding onto the floor. Now I didn't have any clear floor space to run away. The next shot he took was at the ceiling fan, and the light there exploded us both into darkness. It was around 6 PM, so we had some light from outside the window, but that was about it! He took a third shot at my computer screen, again sending more glass shards to the floor, and the fourth shot nearly hit my boyfriend! The super bright flashes of light that the gun rounds released were near blinding, and for a second or two I could not see a thing. Plus, add the fact that this guy just blew out the lights in the room, and I really could see nothing. Next, he placed his left foot through the window!" I asked her, "Then what happened?" She responded, "To protect myself with the little bit of light that was coming from the outside window, I threw a ceramic coffee cup that I had left on my nightstand with the milk I had the night before. I always like to have a nice warm cup of milk with some apple turnovers because that's the only way I can sleep for the night. The meth keeps me up a lot, and I don't want to be super alert all the time either! So, I threw this white cup at the base of his foot, and it hit its target. He was super mad and very aggressively brought his other foot into the room!

He was limping in his Timberland boots and was not happy at all!" I then asked her what happened next. She responded, "He took off his sunglasses and had this devious smile on his face as he raised the rifle in my direction!"

I was terrified as I heard each second of Ms. J's story, recounting this horrifying ordeal. She began, "He pulled the trigger and…" She gushed a ton of tears, crying inconsolably, and I handed her a tissue. She continued, "He pulled the trigger and it was a blank!" He then continued to reload his rifle, but before he closed back the gun..." I reassured her with "Ms. J, it's going to be OK. If you don't want to talk about it, that's perfectly fine." She said, "No, no, telling this story—my story—helps me in coping." I then told her, "Please continue then." So Ms. J stated, "He pulled the trigger for the second time, but suddenly there were police sirens, and he threw down his rifle!" She continued, "Those sirens saved my life that night!"

I asked her, "How are you feeling today?" She was quite resilient after having survived an ordeal like that and responded, "I'm going to make it!" This mental toughness is what it takes to thrive in life, and most certainly it is the correct attitude to possess if one wants to successfully combat any type of drug addiction. I am so glad that she physically survived this ordeal, but that is only the beginning. Physical scars may take two to three weeks to heal, but emotional trauma can take as much as thirty, forty years and more to heal. However, I pray with her and know that it is the power of God that can truly restore her back to completeness. At the addiction level, I offer pharmacotherapy that helps people deal with the cravings of drug dependence when those addicted to crystal methamphetamine are trying to come clean, but there are wounds that run deep—way deeper than the human eye can behold. It is sort of a spiritual hollow-point bullet trajectory through the human body. It may make a pin-hole entry, but inside, it leaves a totally obliterated trail of abject destruction.

Crystal methamphetamine can be smoked, snorted, and injected and can give its user a sense of absolute euphoria, domination, and boundless energy. The high lasts approximately five to ten hours but can go as long as an entire day and night. Methamphetamine generates its effects by increasing the amount of dopamine produced by the brain.

Let me delve into more detail about dopamine. It does not matter whether you snort, smoke, or take methamphetamine intravenously; it will end up in your blood and eventually get into your brain! Not good. Let me explain why. The molecular shape, size, and chemical composition is very similar to dopamine, which is more than happy to work on each brain cell/nerve cell called a neuron. The brain is made up of hundreds of billions of these nerve cells, which have three main parts: a cell body that contains the nucleus and hence the genetic material; dendrites, or short fibers, that receive messages from other neurons and relay them to the cell body; and an axon, a long single fiber that carries messages from the cell body to dendrites of other neurons. The axons of one neuron and the dendrites of a neighboring neuron are very close to one another, yet they do not actually touch. Therefore, to communicate with each other, they use chemical messengers called neurotransmitters. When one neuron wants to send a message to its fellow neuron, it releases a neurotransmitter from its axon into a small space called a synapse that separates the two nerve cells. The neurotransmitter crosses the synapse and attaches to specific places on the dendrites of the next neuron called receptors. Once the neurotransmitter has relayed its message, it is either destroyed or taken back into the first neuron, where it is recycled for use the next time around. There are several different neurotransmitters, but the one most influenced by methamphetamine is dopamine. It is the pleasure neurotransmitter. This neurotransmitter is released when we eat chocolate, make a good friendship, skydive, go on a roller coaster, eat a juicy steak or delicious coconut-glazed salmon, and so on. When something pleasurable happens, certain axons release a considerable amount of dopamine, which attaches to receptors on the neighboring neurons of dendrites' and passes on the pleasure sensation. This pleasure ends when the dopamine released from the receptors is pumped back into the neuron that released it at first.

Usually neurons recycle Dopamine; however, methamphetamine can mimic dopamine, and the neurons take up the methamphetamine; once it is inside the neuron, it makes the neuron release boatloads of dopamine. This extra dopamine makes the individual feel intense pleasure ALL day long. However, all of these pleasurable feelings do not last forever and are followed by all those unpleasant cravings or by a "crash." Methamphetamine also affects other neurons that contain the neurotransmitters serotonin and norepinephrine! The half-life of meth is around twelve hours, meaning that 50 percent of the drug is cleared from your body in about twelve hours, and it is still not 100 percent gone after that. If taken intravenously with a needle, the half-life is still around twelve hours; smoking and snorting it is a shorter half-life. If meth is smoked, elimination from the body takes approximately three days. Additionally, for an older individual, it takes longer to be eliminated from the body. The compound resveratrol decreases the release of dopamine and the hyperactivity of crystal methamphetamine use. Some studies point to Rivastigmine and Wellbutrin to reduce cravings for methamphetamine. There are also vaccines that bind methamphetamine in the body and block its stimulating and euphoric effects. For cravings, Resveratrol is found in blueberries, raspberries, and cranberries.

Some addicts take methamphetamine every few hours for days! This is why Ms. J went through $1,000 a day for her habit. I asked Ms. J, “Didn’t you think about how much your drug habit was costing you?” She responded, “I didn’t really consider the cost. I was so addicted to it that I ‘just’ had to have it, no matter what!” The short-term effects are decreased appetite, increased wakefulness, faster breathing, rapid and irregular heartbeat, and increased blood pressure and body temperature. These patients can have fevers of 103 degrees, “just out of the blue,” as many of them have confessed to me. In that case, the first question I have for them is, “Are you abusing methamphetamine?” Some are honest with me and hang their head in shame; I do not judge any of them. The ones who tell me the truth are the individuals that I can truly help.

The ones that lie to me are so much harder to reach. One such patient is Ms. Taj. Ms. Taj comes in with her famous one-liners like, "Well, Dr. Alexis, I can tell that you work out!" I respond, "Thanks, but your urine screen is dirty for illicit drugs." Ms. Taj responds, "Doc, that can't be possible. I'm clean. I don't hang with that kind of crowd anymore!" Little does Ms. Taj realize that I have the confirmation from labs that proves she abuses at least two grams of heroin daily with Xanax, crystal meth, and cocaine. Like I said, her drug screen is dirty—super dirty. For her to lie to me is hurtful, as I want EVERY patient to be successful here at our center. But the main person Ms. Taj is lying to is herself. There is something about being honest with someone else than with yourself; it opens the door for recovery. When we have group counseling, it is critical that our patients go to these meetings, as I let many of them know that we do not run a pill mill here! If they are not up for counseling, after three missed sessions, they are shown the front door. We want total commitment at our center at all times.

Now, let us get back to methamphetamine for a minute. Manufacturers make most of the meth found in the United States in "superlabs," and often in Mexico. Others make meth in clandestine labs with inexpensive over-the-counter ingredients found in cold medicines. To counter this, the Drug Enforcement Administration (DEA) requires pharmacies to keep a purchase record of products containing pseudoephedrine.

Long-term risks of methamphetamine in people injecting it include HIV, hepatitis C, and hepatitis B. Being on methamphetamine alters a person's judgment and behavior, leading to unsafe sexual practices. Additionally, methamphetamine may worsen the progression of HIV/AIDS with its consequences. Clinical studies have shown that HIV causes more injuries to nerve cells of the human body and even more cognitive deficits in people with HIV who abuse methamphetamine. Methamphetamine also rots away the teeth, and I have seen many patients abusing methamphetamine that had dental abscesses and severe pulpitis with horrific jaw line recession. This drug will literally eat your face away! People abusing methamphetamine are also prone to hallucinations (seeing and/or hearing things that do not exist in reality). A 2009 report from the RAND Corporation observed that methamphetamine abuse cost the United States 23.4 billion dollars in 2005 alone. Additionally, abusers of this drug are paranoid and do not trust their own mothers and fathers.

One of my patients, Mr. Seth, was a chronic methamphetamine user for the past ten years, and thus was extremely hyper. He usually wore a white and blue polo shirt with blue jeans that had holes in them at the knees. He would pace the floor in the examination room at least 100 times. I would greet him quite amicably with a "Good morning, Mr. Seth, how …" He would then jump right in before I could even finish greeting him, with a, "It's a GREAT, GREAT, GREAT MORNING, DOC. THERE'S NO REASON TO EVER HAVE A DOWN DAY! DOC, THE DAY IS WHAT YOU MAKE IT AND YOU GOTTA STAY POSITIVE AND …" I would quickly jump into the fast-flowing verbal Kung Fu match with Mr. Seth, knowing all too well that if I did not speak fast, I would never get the chance to speak at all. The one good thing about being a native New Yorker is that I could match the verbal speed of Mr. Seth and talk as fast as a used-car salesman on steroids without biting my tongue and cheeks—so as to carry on a meaningful conversation with him. As I spoke with Mr. Seth, he nodded his head up and down in a rhythmic fashion, and I certainly did not hear any music playing at all whatsoever! I leaned in closer to Mr. Seth to look at his eardrums, to see if he had an iPod or some small Bluetooth device that was playing music, but I saw no such device! I asked Mr. Seth, "I see you are nodding your head up and down and tapping your feet." Seth responded, "Yes, sir!" I said to him, "Where is your musical device?" He simply responded, "It's a GREAT, GREAT, GREAT MORNING, DOC. THERE'S NO REASON TO EVER HAVE A DOWN DAY! DOC, THE DAY IS WHAT YOU MAKE IT AND YOU GOTTA STAY POSITIVE AND SMILE!" He repeated this no matter what I said. After listening to his heart and lungs and completing my clinical exam, he smiled at me from ear to ear, and I was at least happy that he was jubilant during my extremely mundane examination. His eyes were as wide as a person watching a horror movie yet smiling from ear to ear! It was truly an amazing sight. He usually bit his nails in between pacing back and forth the examination room, as it was nearly impossible for him to simply sit on the examination table. He twisted his head to around 270 degrees Fahrenheit, bit his nails, looked at me and smiled, dropped his hands to his sides, and then repeated this motion with effortless orchestration. Again, as I asked my next question of how he was enjoying counseling, he smiled from ear to ear, nodded his head as if he was listening to music, tapped his feet interjecting this with a rotating head motion and moving it left to right then right to left—to 270 degrees on each side—where he would then proceed to bite his nails, dart a fast smile at me, and drop his hands to his sides.

I enjoyed my time with Mr. Seth; I put my Littman's cardiology stethoscope around my neck and extended my hand to shake his hand, at which he threw out his hand more quickly than a group of kids leaving their last class at the last hour on the last day of school for summer vacation. He held my hand as firm as a grizzly bear coil spring trap, and I thought that I had lost my hand and arm in this hand-shaking frenzy! I simply took one foot back and released my hand with all my strength, smiled, and ran for the door! While I walked backward, he was still holding onto my right hand for dear life and I threw my left hand behind me; I was so desperate to reach the door, with Mr. Seth grinning from ear to ear. I got hold of the metallic doorknob with my left hand, and I knew that I would soon be home, free! I said, "Mr. Seth, it's been great seeing you to—" but before I could get the words out of my mouth, he vehemently erupted, "It's a GREAT, GREAT, GREAT MORNING, DOC. THERE'S NO REASON TO EVER HAVE A DOWN DAY! DOC, THE DAY IS WHAT YOU MAKE IT AND YOU GOTTA STAY POSITIVE AND SMILE!" With the doorknob in my left hand, I now had a secure anchor in place. With all my strength, I fastened my grip on the doorknob, as if my life depended on it, and put my hips and butt synchronously in one sweeping motion and was out of that examination room! I looked down at my sides, ensuring that I had both my arms still attached to my torso and was relieved to see that I did.

He had recently tested positive for methamphetamine use despite being warned about its effects. In addition, he did have one DOWN DAY. He affirmed to me, "Doc, it's not going so well. I spilled coffee on myself not once but twice!" At this moment, he was smiling ear to ear and said, "Well, Doc, I Guess THE DAY IS WHAT YOU MAKE IT AND YOU GOTTA STAY POSITIVE AND SMILE." Those jeans are in fashion today, but when I was growing up, back in the '70s and '80s, kids did not think of that type of jeans as a style at all. Where I came from, they would throw rocks at people they did not like based solely on the way those people dressed. It is a sad state of affairs when people treat you differently just based on aspects of your outer appearance, such as clothes, jewelry, or makeup.

I did not truly realize how methamphetamine could really contain people in that state of not only overdrive but also “hyperdrive.” There is also increased risk of developing Parkinson’s disease from abusing methamphetamine, and yes, if you are around someone who is smoking methamphetamine, although you have never abused it yourself, you will still test positive and lose the job of a lifetime when they test you on the first day of employment. So, young people, be very SELECTIVE with the company you keep.

Despite giving Mr. Seth numerous chances to come clean—nine to be precise—he failed another drug test and had to be released from our program. We made an adequate referral for him to be treated elsewhere. Trying to keep cool with the wrong crowd for just five minutes can bring you severe, bitter repercussions lasting for the next fifteen years! I have seen this numerous times. Therefore, I not only request you, young people, but BEG you to PLEASE be SELECTIVE with the company you keep. You are so much better than those. No one needs to approve of you if you have not approved of yourself first. You have to know the inner you before any individual on the OUTSIDE can even begin to approve of you! The most important component of you is your soul, a component of you that is totally invisible to anyone else. Your height, skin color, weight, gender, national origin, and so forth, are all pale in comparison to your very soul. S.O.U.L. stands for Spirit Overlooking Universe Limitlessly.

I had another patient who had been on methamphetamine; he was not as friendly as Mr. Seth and was quite the paranoid type. Mr. Chad was quite a character. One day, I saw several patients on my list and then looked over the list, and certainly, Mr. Chad was scheduled next for me to see. I knocked on the door of room #1, opened it, and there was Mr. Chad looking at me very suspiciously without blinking his eyes the whole time, while pacing the floor back and forth non-stop. He was about five-foot-two inches tall, with blond hair and blue eyes, and he looked at me from head to toe extremely cautiously. His eyes would also simultaneously dart from the east side of the examination room to the west side at least ten times before he would even speak to me. His hands were in his pockets, while simultaneously he would grind his teeth with his jaw shifting from right to left in a rhythmic motion, like a bull chewing grass while eyeing the farmer suspiciously, not knowing if the farmer was coming closer to make him into his T-bone dinner for the evening meal! I greeted him with a "Good morning, Mr. Chad, how are you doing today?" He responded with a terse "Good." He continued to look at me very suspiciously, and I reviewed his drug screen test results with him. I began, "Mr. Chad, I would love to go over your results with you." He looked at me square in the eye and uttered an extremely slow "OK." I continued, "Your urine drug screen is positive!" He rolled his eyes upward and gave a devious grin while walking to the left side of the room, then the right, eyeing me the whole time in the process. He began the walk again to the right side of the room, now to the left. He leaned against the examination table and said, "Positive, for what?" I explained, "Sir, there is no reason for you to raise your voice." "I'm not raising my voice!" he responded. I told him bluntly, "You are testing positive for crystal methamphetamine." Mr. Chad replied, "I don't know how it got there, Doc. Just don't know!" He then turned his back to me and started pacing around the room.

He was one of our more noncompliant cases, as no matter what we did to help him it just did not seem to work. Mr. Chad had a history of domestic violence, as he had fractured his girlfriend's ribs on the right side, who also had been abusing crystal methamphetamine and heroin for the past ten years. Mr. Chad went on to fail several more drug screens and got kicked out of our program, as he felt the rules applied to all the other patients at our center except for him! He even had the audacity to come back to our clinic for drug treatment after he was officially dismissed. He would yell outside the building, "I want to see the f—ing doctor!" I was not there when he was saying all this, as it was my day off. He was also spotted by staff placing his hands down his pants and touching inappropriate parts of his body while in public.

We eventually did see him again—in the newspaper. Unfortunately, he was arrested after breaking and entering a private residence, which being a felony, he was going to have to do hard time for. One day, a coworker showed me something on her cell phone that I did not want to see, as we work so hard with every patient that comes through our front doors on Whitestick Street. Mr. Chad was arrested as he was a suspect in several neighborhood robberies. I felt bad for Mr. Chad, as I wish for all our patients to succeed in our outpatient program, but this will should also be present on the patient's part to want to be successful.

Another client, Mr. Port, came to our addiction treatment center and, I must say, he was as tall as a skyscraper! Standing six feet ten inches, he was sweating up a storm, had a pulse of 120, with blood pressure 160/110, goose bumps all over his body, bloodshot eyes, and a runny nose. His plaid blue and white short-sleeve shirt was drenched to the point you could see his T-shirt underneath his outer shirt. He had abused crystal methamphetamine, heroin, cocaine, and a number of other drugs. After stabilizing Mr. Port and offering him some juice and directing a portable fan toward him to cool him down, as his temperature was 101 degrees, I asked him several questions. I started with, "Mr. Port, how old are you?" "I am twenty-five years old, Doc" was his response. "What drugs did you use, sir?" He replied, "Cocaine, methamphetamine, heroin." I then asked, "For how long?" He responded, "For at least three years." He then went on to mention, "I'm so ashamed of myself and how low I've descended. I'm doing this program for my mother. She would have never dreamed I'd go this low. I just, just feel so ashamed of myself!" He looked down at the floor, and his sweat was dripping profusely on the russet brown carpet. Drip, drip, drip. It loudly plopped on the ground, just rolling off in waves from his massive six foot ten inch, 300-pound frame. He continued, "I used to play football and had a scholarship to play at WVU." I felt real bad for him, so I asked, "What changed that?" Mr. Port responded, "Well, Doc, I was a straight 'A' student in high school, but despite that, I started to hang out with the wrong crowd." His brown hair was now drenched from all his sweating, and he fixed his eyes downward at the blue carpet situated three feet below him. The sweat from his brown hair dropped onto his upper lip that was quivering, with his massive shoulders trembling. I calmly told him, “Go on.” “Well, these kids were so cool and they wanted to hang out with me. Who would have thought?!” he gushed. With a lot of my patients who have had severe physical or sexual abuse, I find that 99.9 percent of them just want to be accepted by their peer group.

Anyway, we got Mr. Port stabilized and he was not sweating as much now; his temperature came down to 98.9 degrees; and his blood pressure and pulse also stabilized. When Mr. Port was started on Suboxone, he was much calmer, without sweating. Before starting Suboxone, we use the Clinical Opiate Withdrawal Scale (COWS) Assessment. It works like this: there are eleven items I assess as a physician. I want to give you a select peek into how I assess each individual patient before starting the patient on any medications at our treatment facility. The first modality that I assess is the resting pulse. This is in beats per minute after the patient has been quietly resting for one minute. If their pulse rate is 80 or below, they score a zero. Let us look at some clinical cases where the pulse rate is below 80. If the pulse rate is below 60, for example, this can be either good or bad. Let us look at the good first. In well-conditioned endurance athletes, some heart rates have been known to drop to 35 beats per minute due to enhanced vagus nerve activity. Some athletes brag about having a low heart rate, BUT it may not always be a good thing. In an article by Bethany Brookshire, she mentions a study by a cardiac physiologist, named Alicia D'Souza, of the University of Manchester, who made a discovery in the "funny channels" of the sinoatrial node of the heart. The slow heart rate has fewer channels to transmit current through which it controls the activity of heart cells. This is not good! D'Souza focused on ion channels called "HCN4." These HCN4 channels are integral components of sinoatrial node tissue. Endurance training such as the ones that ultra-marathoners undergo may remodel the heart and alter the number of funny channels.

Let us look at another condition that can cause an abnormally low heart rate, giving a zero on the COWS: sick sinus syndrome. In the sick sinus syndrome, the heart's natural pacemaker—the sinoatrial node—is old or diseased. Patients have symptoms of fatigue, lightheadedness, and passing out. The most common cause of sick sinus syndrome is the replacement of sinus node tissue with fibrous tissue. Sometimes, there is an involvement of this fibrosis with lower parts of the heart's electrical conduction system. Let us look at the two systems that control the sinoatrial node. First, there is parasympathetic input via the vagus nerve that tends to slow the heart rate. Second, there is the sympathetic nervous system that tends to speed up the sinoatrial node. Now, let us look at medications that can slow the activity of the sinoatrial node. There are beta-blockers (medications taken for hypertension), Digoxin (a medicine used for congestive heart failure), and Aricept (a medication used to treat Alzheimer's). Other diseases can cause sick sinus syndrome by impacting the shape and functionality of the sinoatrial node. These causes include rheumatic fever and generalized inflammation of the heart. There is also an issue in the blood supply to the sinoatrial node. If a patient has cholesterol plaque buildup in their right or left coronary artery, this can alter the functioning of the heart's sinoatrial node. The right coronary artery in 60 percent of cases supplies blood to the sinoatrial node, and in 40 percent of cases, it is the left coronary artery. Around 5 percent of patients that have suffered a heart attack have reversible sinoatrial node slowing. In one study of forty-six patients with a prior heart attack (twenty-three patients with and twenty-three patients without sick sinus syndrome), the internal heart rate was abnormal in all those patients who had more than a 75 percent narrowing of the sinoatrial node artery but only around 33 percent in those patients with a 50 percent narrowing. In some cases of sick sinus syndrome, the heart can actually speed up. Several risk factors are associated with developing sick sinus syndrome, such as higher body mass index, hypertension, and a prior heart attack. However, advancing age is the most important risk factor for developing sick sinus syndrome. If a patient's pulse rate is between 81 and 100, they score a one on this component. If their pulse rate is between 101 and 120, they score a two. However, if their pulse rate is greater than 120, then they score a four. In these instances, I ensure that they do not have an underlying cardiac condition or metabolic syndrome that can be causing this fast heart rate. If they have hyperthyroidism, this is one major cause of a much quicker heart rate that can throw this testing off.

Let us look at hyperthyroidism for a moment here. Symptoms of hyperthyroidism include anxiety, weakness, tremors, heart racing, heat intolerance, and weight loss despite an increasing appetite. The size of the thyroid gland depends upon the cause of hyperthyroidism. Thyroid size can be massive in Grave's disease or toxic multinodular goiter. Patients with silent thyroiditis may not even have a goiter.

Let us now move on to lab tests to make the diagnosis. Patients generally have a low TSH (thyroid stimulating hormone) level. You also need to look at serum-free T4 and T3. In hyperthyroidism, the free T4 as well as the T3 levels are elevated. Let us look at how to treat hyperthyroidism. A medication called methimazole is used for treatment and is dosed once daily. If a female patient is pregnant, I usually use Propylthiouracil during the first trimester, as fewer risks of birth defects are seen. A patient with a small goiter (swelling of the thyroid gland) and with free T4 (Thyroxine) levels between one and one-and-a-half times the upper limit of normal can be started on 5–10 milligrams once a day. Patients that have free T4 levels between one-and-a-half and two times the upper limit of normal can be started on 10–20 milligrams daily. Patients with large goiters and much more severe hyperthyroidism, that is, free T4 levels two or three times the upper limits of normal, can be started on 20–40 milligrams once a day. Sometimes therapy on methimazole may last for decades.

Let us look at another treatment option for hyperthyroidism—radioiodine ablation. What is the process for radioiodine ablation, you may wonder. The radioiodine is administered as a capsule or oral solution of sodium I-131, which is quickly absorbed from the GI tract and concentrated in the thyroid tissue. Radioiodine induces extensive tissue changes within the thyroid, halting its activities of oversecreting active thyroid hormones. Up to 20 percent of patients fail the first radioiodine treatment and require a second dose. After the radioiodine treatment, all patients must be monitored for swinging in the opposite biochemical direction—to hypothyroidism. Most patients will have normalization of thyroid tests between one and three months. If the patient has a normal functioning thyroid for around six months, TSH is measured from six- to twelve-month intervals for life, as we must closely monitor for an underperforming thyroid, i.e., hypothyroidism. If a patient becomes hypothyroid, synthroid can be started, with the dose of synthroid adjusted to maintain a normal free T4 level. Once a patient's thyroid tests are normal on a stable dose of synthroid, the TSH can be measured once a year. The main test that I usually look at to follow the treatment of hyperthyroidism is the blood's free T4 levels.

Nonetheless, TSH is unreliable; it can remain low for weeks or even for months. When both TSH and free T4 are low, measurement of the blood's T3 is required to distinguish between persistent hyperthyroidism (T3 elevated) and temporary central hypothyroidism (T3 normal or low), which is classically associated with the recovery of brain from radioiodine treatments. Supraventricular tachycardia or atrial tachycardia can also increase the heart rate. You may ask what can be done to address these two cardiac conditions. Well, there are certain approaches I can take as a healthcare professional. I can rub the place where the carotid artery is, and this can slow down the heart rate to its natural rate. However, what if this does not work? In that case, I can gently press on the eyeballs, which is known as the oculocardiac reflex, which coordinates with nerve cells from the eye, communicating with the vagus nerve, which then communicates with the cardiac centers of the human brain stem, leading to decreased output by the sinoatrial node of the heart, i.e., the heart's natural pacemaker. This will slow down the heart and will allow getting the patient's natural heart rate. If this still does not work, the patient can try squeezing his/her nostrils shut while blowing wind through the nose, which usually helps bring down a fast heart rate.

Let us look at supraventricular tachycardia (SVT) for a moment. Usually, SVT can start and stop suddenly; it is caused by a problem with the heart's electrical system. SVT starts in the upper chamber of the heart—the atria. The fast heartbeat can last from several minutes to several hours, which can be terrifying. However, on average, it lasts for 10–20 minutes. In many cases, it happens when you are at rest; in a minority of cases, exercise can trigger it. There are three types of SVT: 1) atrioventricular nodal reentry tachycardia (AVNRT), 2) atrioventricular reentry tachycardia (AVRT), and 3) atrial tachycardia. Symptoms include feeling dizzy, lightheaded, and tired. If, at any time, you feel chest pain or cannot breathe, you MUST dial 9-1-1. The tests that are done include an EKG. Other tests are wearing the Holter monitor, which records the heart's electrical activity over 24–48 hours. With the Holter monitor, you will have electrodes stuck to your chest, which are connected to wires leading to the monitor. You must keep the device and the electrodes dry at all times. Other tests include the event monitor. This device is smaller than a Holter monitor and does not record all the time. When you feel that your heart is skipping a beat or dizzy, press a button on this handheld device attached to your chest, as that may be an underlying indicator that a cardiac event is occurring. This event monitor is worn for thirty days instead of just one or two!

Patients with atrioventricular nodal reentrant tachycardia (AVNRT), who have extremely low pressure, are shocked with the paddles that you see (direct cardioversion). If patients with AVNRT with low pressure, angina, and heart failure, have an IV line in place, they should first receive IV adenosine (6 mg) rather than the aforementioned shock! This is critical to understand. Even before getting adenosine, you want to employ valsalva maneuvers. You may ask how this is done. The patient is placed on his/her back and is asked to take a deep breath first and then exhale with all of his/her might with a closed mouth for 10–15 seconds. Signs that the patient is doing this forcefully enough include distended neck veins, increased tone in the belly muscles, and a flushed face.

Let us look at another technique that we can employ to slow down a fast heart rate before using adenosine medication. There is something called the carotid sinus massage. It was documented in as early as the 18th century and involves putting pressure on the carotid sinus in the neck so as to stimulate the vagus nerve (a parasympathetic nerve). However, later studies showed that distinct nerve fibers are present in the carotid sinus that go to the medulla (part of the brain stem that controls breathing and pulse rate). You may ask, "Where is the crated sinus located?" If you place an index finger of a respective hand on the same side of the neck, for the left side, you would use the left index finger, and for the right side, the right index finger. So, touch the lowest portion of your earlobe—where you put an earring—using your left index finger. Now, go down roughly four inches and then move the index finger forward by approximately half an inch. There you have it, folks! That is the carotid sinus. You have struck gold! You can at least save the life of someone who might be having an extremely fast heartbeat. You want to hold onto that spot firmly for 5–10 seconds. If you are in a hospital setting, medical professionals will check vital signs before and after the maneuver. The heart will be continuously monitored, and a 12-lead EKG will also be done.

Now let us look at contraindications to doing the carotid sinus massage. If a person has had a stroke within the past three months, it is a no-go to; if a patient has had a TIA, it is also a no-go to. You may ask here, “What is a TIA?” A TIA is a transient ischemic attack, which was originally defined as a sudden onset of focal neurologic symptoms lasting less than 24 hours and caused by reversible but lack of blood supply to the brain. However, having said this, there is a risk of permanent tissue damage even when focal neurologic symptoms last less than one hour. There are other conditions that can cause a fast heart rate, such as being anemic. If there is not enough vitamin C in your diet on a daily basis, your body will not be able to take up iron. You need a minimum of 90 milligrams of iron every day if you are a male and 75 milligrams if you are a female. However, if you are a breastfeeding woman, you need 45 milligrams of iron more every day to meet the requirement of 120 milligrams of vitamin C every day in this case. Similarly, if you are a pregnant woman, you need 85 milligrams. One-day- to six-month-old babies generally require 40 milligrams of vitamin C. For our precious little ones going through the terrible twos or, in my son's case when he was two—the Tornadoe Twos, where he was into everything and sometimes would get a scrape here and there—15 milligrams is recommended. Vitamin C is a critical part of the diet and is used to make collagen, which is an important protein used in wound healing. Vitamin C is also needed for the immune system to function properly. It protects our body against free radicals, which have been linked to cancer. In line with cancer, I would like to note that if you are a smoker, you need to add an additional 35 milligrams of vitamin C to your diet! Vitamin C is a water-soluble vitamin, meaning that you will not get its toxic buildup in the body. Excess doses are simply excreted by the kidneys and through the urine. B-complex vitamins are the other water-soluble vitamins. One of the critical B vitamins is vitamin B9 (folate), which is vital for babies' proper neurological development and for an adult, as it can decrease the risk of colon cancer! Coming back to vitamin C, an orange typically has 69 milligrams of vitamin C. Strawberries have 84 milligrams of vitamin C and are also rich in potassium, which helps in lowering blood pressure and magnesium. Strawberries also are rich in the mineral manganese, which can regulate PMS symptoms and help control the uptake of calcium, giving us stronger bones. If you are deficient in manganese, you can have tremors, memory loss, high cholesterol, muscle spasms, a fast heart rate, and osteoporosis. Papayas have 88 milligrams of vitamin C and are great in regulating cholesterol levels. They are also great as a paste for facial massages in that the fruit can remove dead skin. Papayas can also help relieve toothaches and are useful at relieving constipation. Another food that provides an excellent source of vitamin C is kale, at 80 milligrams. Kale is rich in quercetin and kaempferol, which has cardioprotective, antihypertensive, antidepressant, and anticancer properties. {Resume}One study even showed that daily consumption of kale juice for twelve weeks increased HDL (the good cholesterol) by 27 percent and lowered LDL (the bad cholesterol) by 10 percent. One study also showed that steaming kale increased its bile acid-binding effects to 43 percent more to that of cholestyramine—an agent that lowers triglycerides. Do you want to have excellent eyesight as you age? I know I sure do! Kale is rich in lutein and zeaxanthin, which lower cataract and macular degeneration (loss of your central vision).

Next, there are pineapples, which contain 79 milligrams

of vitamin C. Pineapples contain bromelain, which is anticancer and antiarthritic. Let us look at bromeliad for a moment. Did you ever have one of those colds that produce thick, gelatin-like phlegm that you cannot get out? Well, bromelain, a unique enzyme, is associated with a reduction of phlegm that can often build up in the nose, lower throat, and sinuses. Additionally, this same bromelain stimulates protein breakdown, aids in digestion, and treats constipation and diarrhea. Pineapple gives bulk to stools, which helps treat diarrhea and irritable bowel syndrome. Let us quickly look at manganese that is also found in pineapples. Manganese is essential for a critical enzyme in the human body called superoxide dismutase, which takes up free radicals that can ordinarily induce cancer. Another such nutrition-rich fruit is kiwi. It has been native to China for centuries but was only introduced to the United States in the early 1960s. Kiwi has 154 percent vitamin C and is a great sleep inducer. I suggest having 2–3 kiwi fruits one hour before going to sleep. Kiwi has an enzyme known as actinidain that can dissolve proteins. It helps digest protein in the human diet and can be used while suffering from irritable bowel syndrome. Kiwi has vitamins B6, B12, E, A; calcium; potassium; and magnesium, which all help with blood circulation, thereby preventing clots, combating stress, promoting healthy bones and teeth, and maintaining good blood pressure. Kiwi is alkaline and combats all acidic foods, and vitamins C and E are great for the skin. Kiwi also contains omega-3 fatty acids and polyphenols that promote good cardiac health. Kiwi can reduce triglycerides by 15 percent, and it is a safer alternative to an aspirin that can, in fact, cause intestinal bleeding. Kiwi also reduces macular degeneration in older adults. A recent study showed that it is safe from a lot of pesticide residues. Not all kiwi fruits are brown and fuzzy! There is also a variety, the golden kiwi, which has a smooth bronze skin and tastes sweeter. However, kiwi does contain oxalates, which are commonly found in kidney and gallbladder stones, so if you have a history of either of these two conditions, I would suggest you to proceed with kiwi slowly. If you have a family history of kidney or gallbladder stones, I would extend the same precaution!

Mango is the last fruit we will consider that has more vitamin C than an orange. It clocks in at 122.3 milligrams of fully loaded vitamin C. It contains fisetin, gallic acid, astragal, and isoquercitrin, which fight colon, breast, leukemia, and prostate cancers. It lowers cholesterol through a soluble fiber known as pectin. Like kiwi, mango is also alkaline and maintains the body's balance with all the acidic foods that we consume. Mango helps optimize insulin levels in the blood. I recommend boiling mango leaves in water, allowing the mixture to soak overnight, and consuming it in the morning.

Next, let us look at the second criterion of the eleven

items on the COWS scale. It is sweating over the past half hour that is not accounted for by room temperature or patient activity. This is the sweating that occurs with withdrawal from opioids. A patient scores a zero if there is no report of chills or flushing. If the patient has a subjective feeling of chills or flushing, then the score is one. If I, as the clinician physician, observe flushing of the face or moistness, then the score is two. If the patient is simply drenched in sweat on the forehead or another part of the face, the score is three. If the sweat is coming off the face in pools, the score is four! Let us look at the causes of excess sweating. Diabetes can cause excess sweating because when your blood glucose goes to critical lows owing to prior insulin administration and the body releases epinephrine—also known as adrenaline—which causes the release of glucagon (the stored form of glucose from the liver) to counteract the lower blood glucose levels. Epinephrine causes one to sweat. You may ask how do we even begin to make a diagnosis of diabetes. The answer is a fasting blood glucose of greater than or equal to 126. Another method is to look at a test called a hemoglobin A1C. However, before looking at the test, we must first know what hemoglobin is. Hemoglobin is an iron-containing oxygen-transporting protein in the red blood cells. Hemoglobin is the guy, so to speak, that carries oxygen from our right and left lungs to the rest of our body. It also transports carbon dioxide, which is exhaled with each breath that we take. Now, let us get back to hemoglobin A1C. This specific form of hemoglobin measures the 3-month average blood glucose concentration. Why three months? The life of an average blood cell is 120 days, i.e., four months. Glucose molecules can attach to hemoglobin, and this blood HbA1C is then measured. Any HbA1C greater than or equal to 6.5 is diagnostic for diabetes, but this test is generally retested in twenty-four hours. Another test for diabetes is a 2-hour plasma glucose greater than or equal to 200 during a two-hour oral glucose tolerance test. This test is done by not eating or drinking anything for 8–14 hours before the test. Then, the patient must drink a liquid that has 75 grams of glucose. The blood is drawn before drinking the liquid and two more times every sixty minutes after drinking the liquid. If it is greater than or equal to 200, it is also diagnostic for diabetes. The other diagnostic modality for diabetes is random blood glucose of 200 or greater with symptoms of blurred vision, headaches, nausea, vomiting, or feeling that you are about to pass out.

Let us look at other causes of excess sweating that I consider to rule out other medical causes of excess sweating that is NOT related to acute illicit drug withdrawals. These other causes are fevers with an unknown origin, malaria, tuberculosis, menopause, leukemia, HIV/AIDS, and generalized anxiety. Let us look at some modalities that can treat excess sweating. There is a procedure known as iontophoresis that utilizes water to pass an electric current to the skin several times during the week for fifteen minutes each session, which is maintained once every two weeks. Another treatment modality is Botox A. A minute portion of this substance is injected with a fine needle into 30–40 regions in each armpit. This can produce up to twelve months of relief from excess sweating. Another treatment for excess underarm sweating is miraDry, which was approved by the FDA in 2011. It utilizes electromagnetic energy that places heat on sweat glands and destroys them. In severe cases, there is a surgery known as thoracic sympathectomy, which cuts the sympathetic nerves responsible for sweating. Complications include excess sweating in other parts of the body and nerve damage. Tuberculosis (TB) can also cause excess sweating. What is TB, you may ask. TB bacteria are spread via the air from one individual with the disease, who coughs, speaks, or sings in public, to another. People in the vicinity, who breathe in these bacteria, can then be infected. TB is not spread through handshakes, by sharing the same food or drink, touching toilet seats, kissing, or sharing toothbrushes. When a person breathes in TB bacteria, the bacteria settle in the lungs and begin to multiply. Then, they move to other parts of the body via the blood stream and can migrate to the brain, kidneys, or spine. TB in the lungs or throat is infectious but that in the kidney or spine is not so.

Let us look at the differing types of TB. There is latent TB and TB disease. Individuals with latent TB infection have the TB bacteria in their bodies, but they are not clinically sick because the bacteria are dormant and not active. This set of people cannot spread the disease to other people, but they may develop TB disease in the future. These people are still provided treatment so that their risk of developing the disease is much lower down the road. Now, let us look at the other group of people that have the TB disease. Persons with TB are sick from the active bacteria that are multiplying and actively destroying tissue in their bodies. These people also usually have the symptoms of TB disease. People with TB disease of the lungs or throat are capable of spreading the bacteria to others and are prescribed medications that treat the disease. You may be wondering what you should do if you have spent time with someone with latent TB infection. A person with latent TB infection cannot spread germs to other people. You do not need to be tested if you have spent time with someone with latent TB infection. However, if you have spent time with someone with TB disease or someone with the symptoms of TB, you must get yourself tested. You may wonder how to get tested for TB. There are two tests to detect TB infection: a skin test and a blood test. The Mantoux tuberculin skin test is done by injecting a small amount of fluid called tuberculin intradermally and is read within 48–72 hours by a certified medical professional. Let us look at how to interpret these skin test results because I have had hundreds of patients throughout the years, who ask me how best to interpret them! After the medical professional injects 0.1 ml or 5 units of the tuberculin, a positive result of greater than or equal to five millimeters swelling on the skin is seen in patients who have HIV infection or risk factors for HIV infection, those have had recent close contact with a person with known active TB, patients with a chest x-ray consistent with prior TB patients with organ transplants, and other immunosuppressed patients (receiving the equivalent of prednisone 15 mg/day for one or more months).

Let us look at those cases wherein within 48 hours, the skin swells to 10 millimeters, which is a positive result for TB. In patients who have immigrated from highprevalence countries, IV drug users, and high-risk congregate settings. Let us go back to treatment regimens: for latent TB based on CDC guidelines, 9 months of INH (Isoniazid) on a daily basis. If patients are known to regularly miss their appointments or have transportation issues, a 6-month course can provide robust protection. However, having said that, treatment modalities less than nine months are not recommended for children or for patients with fibrotic lesions on chest radiographs (CXR). Vitamin B6 supplementation of 25–50 mg every day must be also taken to prevent neuropathy, especially in patients with diabetes, alcoholism, malnutrition, and HIV infection. Let us look at other treatment regimens. There are four months of rifampin, which is less toxic to your liver. Let us look at exactly how isoniazid works to destroy TB. Isoniazid stops the production of a very specific type of acid that makes up the wall of bacteria. Specifically, it is the mycolic acids that make up a bacteria's cell walls that protects the bacteria against hostile forces in the human body's immune system. At therapeutic levels, isoniazid kills TB bacteria BOTH inside human tissue and outside of the tissue. Certain liver tests must be taken while a patient is on isoniazid like AST and ALT levels at baseline before starting this medication and at least monthly. If either the ALT or AST levels increase three to five times above the upper limits of normal, the medication should be stopped, at least temporarily.

Now that we have discussed treatment for the latent phase of TB, let us look at the treatment for active TB. For active TB, there are two phases of treatment—the intensive phase and the continuation phase. Let us start with the intensive phase. The intensive phase includes the drugs isoniazid, rifampin, pyrazinamide, and ethambutol, which are administered to the patient for the first two months. Why are these four drugs necessary, you may ask? Great question! This regimen reduces the risk of secondary resistance to rifampin in regions with a high rate of primary resistance to isoniazid (>4 percent). Once these first two months are completed, a repeat clinician assessment is conducted with repeat chest radiographs and repeat sputum for acid-fast bacilli smear and culture. Patients typically show clinical improvement within days and weeks of starting appropriate treatments.

Now let us consider phase two of the treatment, known as the continuation phase. This is the regimen beyond the first two months and comprises the two medications isoniazid and rifampin. These medications are administered for at least four additional months—for a total of six months. The use of a six-month regimen of rifampin is supported by randomized trials with 1,451 patients with lung TB that compared the effectiveness of six months of isoniazid and rifampin (plus pyrazinamide for the first two months) versus nine months of isoniazid and rifampin. Patients that received the six-month regimen were more likely to complete therapy (61 vs. 51 percent).

Your next logical question may be: Are there cases in which we may have to extend the continuation phase? Great question! The answer is, yes! The continuation phase should be extended to seven months in the following instances: patients have cavitary lung lesions from the tuberculosis bacteria seen on chest radiographs and positive sputum culture after the first two-month intensive phase regimen. Furthermore, the continuation phase is extended to seven months in patients that did not receive an intensive phase regimen that included the two months of pyrazinamide. Previously, we have discussed how isoniazid works in the body. Let us now look at how rifampin works to defend our bodies against the TB bacteria. This medication blocks bacterial genetic growth. Specifically, it stops bacterial RNA synthesis by binding to an enzyme that the RNA needs in working with DNA to produce more active TB.

Let us look at menopause as another cause of sweating. Menopausal symptoms including hot flashes, emotional lability, and vaginal dryness occur, on average, four years prior to the last menstrual period. Up to 80 percent of women experience hot flashes, which can come on very suddenly and result in much drenched clothing. During menopause, women have low estrogen levels and elevated follicle-stimulating hormone concentrations (FSH). In the late reproductive years before the onset of the menopausal transition, serum inhibin A and inhibin B begin to decrease, serum FSH increases, and estradiol levels are preserved. However, luteal phase progesterone levels decrease as fertility potential declines. The first half of the menstrual cycle begins to shorten, going from 14 to 10 days. More irregular menstrual cycles are known for more intense fluctuations in blood FSH levels and estradiol levels. A random blood sample will reveal high FSH and low estradiol concentrations, which is consistent with menopause; however, FSH and estradiol levels may return to the normal premenopausal range. One study showed that a random blood FSH level greater than 25 international units per liter is characteristic of the late menopausal transition, but measurement of serum FSH during the late menopausal transition is not recommended due to its variability. There are also other changes we consider as physicians, for instance, decreases in blood inhibin B hormone levels and the anti-Müllerian hormone (AMH). Additionally, ovarian follicles decrease in overall population. Some of the symptoms of menopause include the following. Hot flashes begin as sudden heat in the chest and then spread to the face rapidly and becomes generalized. The heat sensation lasts around three minutes and is associated with heavy sweating and some palpitations, and can be followed by chills and anxiety. These hot flashes can occur several times a day, and generally last for one year in 80 percent of patients. Hot flashes stop within four to five years of onset; however, in up to 10 percent of women these hot flashes can last into their seventies. Hot flashes are caused by changes that occur in the part of the brain called the hypothalamus as a result of lowered estrogen levels. Premenopausal women physiologically initiate mechanisms to dissipate heat when the core body temperature increases by 0.4 degrees Fahrenheit; however, this mechanism of heat dispersal occurs with much lower increases in menopausal women. The hot flash comes from the improper widening of blood vessels that would ordinarily be constricted with increased blood flow in the skin and hands. Sweating results in a very quick loss of heat and decrease in core body temperature. Shivering occurs as a normal physiological mechanism to restore the core body temperature to normal. Estrogen restores the optimal temperature zone and obliterates the hot flashes. Hormonal therapy with estrogen and progesterone (to decrease risk factors for uterine cancer) can be administered. Special caution should be extended to women that have a history of breast cancer, coronary heart disease, stroke, and venous blood clots. For example, the medication Bazedoxifene, which is a selective estrogen receptor modulator (SERM) when combined with estrogen As- (estrogen 0.45 mg/bazedoxifene 20 mg), has been shown to decrease hot flashes by 75 percent. Other modalities to treat hot flashes include Effexor, Paxil, Celexa, and Lexapro. Gabapentin is an antiepileptic medication used to treat hot flashes. It also has several clinical indications and can be used for diabetic neuropathy of the feet and the severe neuropathic pain that follows a bout with shingles. Gabapentin at 300 milligrams three times a day has been shown to be quite effective. When hot flashes occur at night, they generally take place in the first four hours of sleep. However, hot flashes are suppressed during REM sleep. Studies have shown that, when women experience hot flashes primarily at night, Gabapentin taken at night results in fewer women being awoken from their sleep. If night sweats do occur, women find they can fall back to sleep more easily after the treatment. At higher doses of Gabapentin, let us say 2,400 milligrams daily when carefully titrated over a two-week period, the effects were similar to receiving estrogen. One caveat is that with dosages of Gabapentin this high, side effects can include nausea and vomiting, headache, dizziness, and altered mental status; therefore, I extend to you this word of caution: be careful! Gabapentin can A) strengthen bones; B) decrease the over proliferation of uterine tissue that leads to the possibility of uterine cancer; and C) have a neutral effect on breast tissue, thereby posing less of a breast cancer risk. Other treatments for hot flashes include Gabapentin Actavis 300mg. Catapres, used for high blood pressure control, can also be used to address symptoms of hot flashes.

Other causes of sweating include brain tumors, spinal cord injuries, Parkinson's disease, multiple sclerosis, and Frey's syndrome (sweating on the cheeks that occurs when an individual eats, visualizes, or dreams about food, which produces powerful salivation). Frey's syndrome is the result of damage to the auriculotemporal nerve during head and neck surgery.

Let us look at a special type of headache that causes sweating, and in this case, I am not referring to migraines. Rather, I am talking about a cluster headache. This type of headache is limited to one side of the face, with severe attacks of pain centered around the eye, the region above the eye, or pain focused in the temples. These attacks can occur up to eight times in a day, with their duration ranging from 15 to 180 minutes. There is a bloodshot eye on one side, eyelid edema on the other side, and nasal congestion or runny nose on the same side as the headache. Moreover, there is a sensation of fullness in the ear, and the eyelids on the affected side tend to droop with a pinpoint pupil, all on the same side where the headache is occurring. Let me discuss treatments for cluster headaches, as the pain can be so severe that people have attempted suicide from an acute attack. Since I am about saving lives—I have a motto: NOT ON MY WATCH, BUDDY!—we start off first by administering 100 percent oxygen by facial mask and then 6 mg of subcutaneous Imitrex. Imitrex works at the molecular level by binding to serotonin receptors in the blood vessels that are in the brain! Amazing, right? This then causes the blood vessels to narrow and reduces neurologically mediated inflammatory responses. Once the Imitrex is injected just under the skin, its onset is around 10 minutes, providing much-needed relief. If for some reason my patient cannot tolerate the injection, then intranasal Imitrex is also available as a 20 milligram formula, and it must be sprayed into the nostril on the opposite side of the headache. The onset of action is slightly longer, taking around 15–30 minutes to kick in.

These are all the medical conditions I mentally go through as possible causes of sweating when I consider a person addicted to opioids who is undergoing active withdrawal! The other nine criteria I look at while assessing opioid withdrawal include restlessness, pupil size, bone or joint aches, runny nose or eyes watering, GI upset, tremors, yawning, anxiety/irritability, and gooseflesh skin. The first two criteria gave you a very brief peek into the way I look at each patient who is addicted to opioids or any other illicit substance, like crystal methamphetamine. The remaining nine are beyond the scope of this book, but I want you to appreciate the sophistication of addiction medicine and the focus that I place on each and every single patient that I clinically evaluate and then administer treat. The patient I talked about earlier, Mr. Port, did well in our program until about three weeks into it. We later read about him too. He was arrested for breaking and entering a private residence. Once again, we treat every human being with dignity, but we cannot jump inside your body and control your actions once you are outside our clinic doors, in your private life. It takes a lot of owning up, to remain in our program. We had a mother and son both in our program for abusing all kinds of illicit drugs. The mother was around 58 and was still in our program after seven months. Her son was in our program up until he thought the rules did not apply to him. We released him after he failed three drug screens.

The mother recently came to our clinic for treatment. I knocked on the door and then entered the examination room and, sure enough, there was Ms. Cee. I said, "Good morning, Ms. Cee!" She responded, "Good morning, Doc." She was wearing a white and brown stripe blouse and seemed like she had recently had a perm done. I continued, "How is your son doing?" She responded, "He was doing well, keeping out of trouble, until you guys kicked him out of the program and now he's in jail. I guess he went off the deep end and... " I cut her statement like a navy submarine cutting through the ice on the sea surface. "Ms. Cee, first of all, we never kick anyone out of our program, and second of all, your son had numerous chances in our program but failed drug screen after drug screen." A lot of the patients in our program have family members that are also in the program. There is this attitude that patients adopt, believing that you do not have to take any responsibility for your actions. This mother thought that was true in this case since it was her son. After I corrected her on this error, she continued, "You are most certainly right, Doc.

You definitely gotta listen to 'em rules!" I responded with an emphatic "That's right!" Her son had been given repeated warnings four weeks earlier about his dirty urine test results, but every time he failed to take ownership of his actions, thinking that it was everyone else's fault except his own. When asked about his dirty urine test results one day, he responded, "Doc, that urine screen is not mine!" I responded, "Well, who do you think it belongs to then?" He replied, "Doc, I just don't know. I really can't tell!" He even went on to say, "Doc, I think you have to look at your lab equipment and check it out!" I look at him incredulously and responded, "I don't know about that, man!" Her son was a soft-spoken man standing six feet two inches tall with thin-rimmed glasses. He had the appearance of a young John Lennon without the beard, and wore a blue baseball cap religiously. He never lost his temper even when he knew that we would be dismissing him from the clinic. He was the type of patient that could have gone on and been an excellent investigative reporter for a national media outlet. He was always inquisitive, and when he looked at you, his gaze would peer deep into your soul and uncover it for what it was! I am sure when he peered deep into my consciousness he saw, as a matter of fact, CARE, which stands for "concerned about resourceful results for everyone."

The reason I mention resourceful results is that there are natural barriers that drug addicts presently have in their day-to-day environment. How do we best overcome natural limitations that are ever present in such an environment? Let us look at examples of some problems that I try to solve with my patients daily: 1) There may be limitations in obtaining transportation to come to the clinic. 2) There may be childcare issues that impede them from coming to our clinic before we close. 3) There may be drug-addicted children of the drug-addicted parent that cause them grief. 4) There may be a child that recently died in the life of the individual currently receiving treatment for their drug addiction. 5) A parent may be currently involved in a custody battle with their ex-spouse. 6) There are often coexisting mental health issues with the patient's drug addiction. 7) There may be a best friend that died from an illicit drug overdose. 8) There may be marital stressors.

We saw one patient that had a jealous brother-in-law who had been kicked out of our program for noncompliance with our guidelines. Again, he felt the rules did not apply to him, so what did he do? He spiked his sister-in-law's food and beverage with some heroin, making her test dirty the next time she came to be drug screened at our clinic. She was released from our program for 30 days. She was in tears. I asked her what happened. She responded, "My brother-in-law—I know he did it. He shoots up all the time!" I walked over and handed her several tissues to wipe her tears, and her cries developed into an all-out, deep, and belly-shaking weeping, the kind that you would have if you lost a child or home or experienced any other major catastrophic life events that could possibly occur to an individual. I responded, “It’s a thirty-day suspension, Ms. V, and it’s not forever. I will taper your medication dose and I’m fighting for you one hundred percent!” Ms. V responded, “Thanks, Doc, I won’t let you down.”

There may be issues of domestic violence as some boyfriends threaten violence against their girlfriends because they see their girl becoming clean, meaning that they (the boyfriends) are no longer needed in the picture. Some boyfriends even see me as the enemy, for as long as they know their girlfriends are addicts, the boyfriends can assert dominance over them!

In a discussion with one woman, she told me that her boyfriend had once kidnapped her and taken her to South Carolina as he wanted to reassert his control over her. He felt as if he was losing his control once he saw that she was becoming clean by visiting my clinic! He had once wielded this control over her endlessly and mercilessly! Subsequently, he was arrested on kidnapping charges. When I saw her, she had scratch marks on her olive-complexioned face, and with tears running down her face she stated, "I'm just glad to be here!" I reviewed with her my CARE model, showing her that it was a way of breaking out and away from this psychotic boy-"friend." I identified her family members that could be a haven for her, especially if she was not comfortable staying at the local neighborhood women's shelter where she would be an easy target for her boyfriend to find. She had relatives at a distant location, and we identified several such relatives that we mutually agreed would be a perfect fit! I am not at liberty to mention which relatives and what states they live in, for obvious reasons, as the anonymity and safety of each of my patients is my top priority! Her parents already saw her as a “lost” cause and refused to help her! Their own daughter—how sad! Tears were starting to form in my own eyes and I had to clear my throat a few times. I had to get a tissue for her and another for myself.

The next time she came to my office, she was all smiles, had applied makeup, and seemed to be in excellent spirits. She was animated as she spoke, “I am going to stay with my…” were the first words out of her mouth when I asked her how she was doing. Two weeks before that she had been weeping inconsolably, drenching her white T-shirt. When I saw her in this despicable state, at the mercy of her boy-“friend,” it was too much even for me to bear! How could you hear these stories emanating from the human soul and not be moved? You surely would have to have a heart of indomitable cold stone, that is how!

Regarding envious boyfriends, it can also swing in

the opposite direction. I had a 300-pound, six foot seven man, Mr. Raj, that was doing well in our program, but who had a possessive girlfriend. She got into frequent fights with him every time he came in for treatment. She was five foot four and 110 pounds with 10 soaking-wet towels on her shoulders. That is how petite she was! Yet she would muster all the energy in that tiny frame to nearly lift him off the ground, as he described it, before he came to our treatment clinic in the morning for his 9:30 appointment and slam him against a wall in their apartment! Mr. Raj added, “Doc, it’s crazy. She is small, and to throw me against the wall, I could never imagine it!” He went on to say, “After she throws me against the wall, her voice changes into a very deep baritone and she hurls the most vile messages that I can’t repeat!” At this point all the hairs on my back had risen, like Lazarus, and I felt more startled than ever before! I could feel the very hairs on my scalp standing tall like soldiers at complete attention. He then proceeded to tell me, “She then throws me on the bed and with superhuman strength takes a pillow and starts to suffocate me!”

This was a patient that had a lower leg infection and possessed limited financial resources, and he felt that he had been neglected by his vascular surgeon because of his financial difficulties. I truly felt bad for this gentle giant of a man. He wore glasses and a dark blue baseball cap. And he would generally converse with pursed lips, which made you savor every word he spoke. With every second of interaction, I wanted to find ways that I could get him help for his lower leg infection. I called in some antibiotic dressings that are known to help debride the dead tissue in chronic wounds and allow the fresh tissue with granulation tissue to be properly laid down.

He continued, “I have to use all of my might to get that pillow off of my face because if I don’t, I know that I’m gonna die!" He related to me, "I finally give the pillow a firm push and twist my hips with all the power that is left in me, and then and only then do I break free, hurling this demon-possessed woman to the ground!"

The day he first came to my clinic, the lower corner of his lip had deep scratch marks and his entire face had sustained least twelve scratch wounds. He had to be placed on antibiotics to prevent severe infection due to all the filthy bacteria that live under the human fingernail. For starters, there are E. coli and Staphylococcus aureus bacteria under fingernails. E. coli is the bacterial agent that can make you have hemorrhagic diarrhea, resulting in possible death. Staphylococcus can cause horrific skin abscesses and pneumonia, and if it is MRSA—a superbug—it can kill you, shutting down your heart brain, kidneys, and other critically vital organs via sepsis—a life-threatening reaction to a severe infection in the human body. MRSA is spread from contact with an infected wound or from sharing personal items like towels, razors, and brushes that have touched infected skin. MRSA infection rates increase when a person is in crowded quarters like school classrooms, military personnel in barracks, daycare, and for those that have recently received any type of inpatient care. Two in every one hundred people carry MRSA. There are steps you can take to reduce your risk of MRSA infection. Maintain good hand hygiene and wash your hands often. You must keep cuts well covered until they have completely scabbed over. You must never share towels and razors. If you work out at the gym, sanitize that weight bench with a Clorox sanitizer wipe. The symptoms of MRSA are bumps that are red, swollen, tender, and full of pus, and in many cases, there is a fever. Treatment includes intravenous vancomycin 20 mg/kg/ dose every eight to twelve hours.

Anyway, Mr. Raj came back to my office in two

months and I examined his leg that had previously been ulcerated. Before I treated this ulcer, you could smell the rotting flesh from at least 200 feet away, and it was the sight of blood mixed with green yellow pus that told me I needed to do something and—fast! When I looked at the wound after Mr. Raj came back, it had totally scabbed over and he remarked, “Doc, this is the best my wounds have looked in over a year!” I had prayed to Jesus to help me select the correct dressing for such a horrific leg wound, and God came through again!

Let us go back for a second to my CARE model. Some patients face limitations regarding transportation to the clinic as they may live two hours away (by car) and simply do not have access to transportation or have anyone that can drive them to the clinic. For example, Mr. Zax once told me, “Doc. I’m sorry I’m late. Can I still be seen?” To which I responded, “Mr. Zax, I will never turn you away, but can you please explain why you are late?” Mr. Zax replied, “I know I’m late—so sorry. What time was I supposed to be here?” I responded, “You were supposed to be here at 9 a.m. today.” Mr. Zax responded, “Oh, Doc, I didn’t know!” He continued, “What time is it now?” I responded, ”3 p.m.” He replied, “Really? You got to be kidding me!” I responded, “Oh no. I wouldn’t be kidding at all!” Mr. Zax said, “Aw, man, it’s that public transportation. They canceled on me at the last minute. I got to get a car soon.” He continued, “I called them at nine in the morning at least two days ahead of time, letting them know that I had to come to your clinic, and you see what they do to me?” I responded to Mr. Zax, “I believe you, man. I wouldn’t doubt you and I’m sure not going to turn you away!” Transportation can be very challenging for some patients that live up to 70 miles away, while other patients just live 100 feet from the center, and so even on the most inclement of days, they still arrive on time.

The winding mountains, terrain, and rockslides do not make the commute any easier for some of the drivers of public transportation. One time when I was driving out of Welch, West Virginia, a rockslide mixed with thick viscous mud had covered the entire road. This mud resembled the red-hot lava from a volcano that is bright red initially and then, as it cools, it becomes dark brown and then black magma. The average temperature of lava is around 1,300–2,400 degrees Fahrenheit. The double solid yellow lines on the mountain road were very faint and seemed to have cracks in them from years of car tires traversing over them. They resembled golden serpents with their twisting configurations, and if you dared to cross over them to overtake a slow-moving vehicle, they would bite you by allowing you to get struck by another car head-on! That was mountain justice coming at you—all for daring to cross that forbidden double yellow line.

Several road crews were positioned strategically that day. They had their orange and blue US Department of Transportation mandated Chevy Tahoes parked perpendicular to the side of the road with their yellow and white lights flashing on top of their hoods, which was blinding to the eye even in daylight! I would look at the light temporarily and close my eyes and WOW! I could still see those flashing lights spinning up a frenzy. I could not believe how those lights would dance to the left, then to the right of my field of vision even after I had closed my eyes for a solid two minutes! It was amazing!

I laughed to myself, and the guy in the opposite lane stared at me strangely. He was driving a Red Ford 350 that was on an eight-inch lift with sparkling chrome hubcaps and rims. He had revved the engine as his truck was in neutral and he did not want to put his foot on his truck's brakes every second. The windshield wiper on his truck was turned to automatic low intermittent speed. I had my window down and he did too. He spoke first, "Man, I'm tired of being stuck here in traffic, but I wish I knew what you are laughing at, because I want to laugh too!" I responded, "Those spinning lights on top of the Department of Transportation SUVs are so bright that I have to close my eyes to spare my vision." This guy began to laugh too and remarked, "That is so true, man!" I continued, "But that's not all. After you close your eyes, you can see the lights dancing on the black screen of your closed eyes from left to right, then upward followed by a downward motion!" He remarked, "That's incredible!" He went on to tell me that when he was at a baseball game where the Los Angeles Dodgers were playing the Cubs, the game was moving so slowly that he would periodically close his eyes. He continued, "It was the bottom of the ninth inning at 10 p.m., and the game was so slow that I closed my eyes and the most beautiful thing happened—a kaleidoscope of figures danced before my eyes in vivid blues and greens, and the tighter I closed my eyes, the faster these figures moved around!" We both simultaneously laughed at this moment. He seemed to be about 45 years old with a blue and gold WVU football cap on, a red shirt, and a coal-dusted face. He had a thick brown beard and a wide smile, and overall seemed pretty good-natured.

His side of the traffic began to slowly move forward, and he put his foot on his accelerator and waved goodbye and went ahead. In the background, you could hear loud police sirens about half a mile away and see their vibrant blue and white flashing lights coming from the East. There were also fire engines approaching from the west with their blaring sirens and flashing red and white lights. The police seemed to effortlessly climb that mountain in their Dodge Charger Pursuit with its V8 engine, 370 horsepower, and 396 lb.-ft of torque. It was like a rocket ship on wheels! Anyway, there were at least

30 cars in front of me and I did not see any use in getting angry. I just played some Alvin Slaughter music and some Brooklyn Tabernacle music to soothe my nerves. The roads were slippery too as it had just rained, and whenever the coal trucks passed through the mountains, they would always drop a little coal onto the treacherous mountains. Sometimes the vehicles would hydroplane, that is, water would get between the tires and separate the truck tires from the road underneath. In a broad highway turn, if the front wheels lose traction, the car will drift toward the outside of the road. If the rear wheels lose traction, the back of the car will go sideways into a skid. If all four wheels lose traction simultaneously, the vehicle will slide in a straight line. As the coal mixed with the rain on the road, an extremely oily residue that was the natural by-product of this mixture was left behind. Metallurgical coal is found here in West Virginia and is used to make steel. But when steel making shifted

overseas from the United States in the 1970s and 1980s, West Virginia's economy took a huge hit.

Anyway, car after truck after cement mixing truck lined the sides of the mountain that day. I did not mind the wait as long as my music was playing from my Toyota 4Runner. We seemed to move an inch per hour that day and, quite frankly, I was not concerned as I did not want my tires to spin on me as we were one thousand feet high up in the mountains. Any wrong move and I would have spun one thousand feet below to my death! As we were getting closer to the Department of Transportation crew that were directing traffic that night, those blinding yellow and white revolving lights were starting to make me feel dizzy. I immediately popped a Pepto-Bismol effervescent tablet into my mouth with my left hand and felt immediate relief.

The truck behind me was a red Ram 1500 and was blasting some country music. I could see his truck in my rearview mirror swaying from side to side to the beat. The driver wore a brown leather cowboy hat and was rhythmically tapping his left pinky, left ring finger, and left middle finger continuously in a sequential fashion on the side door of his truck like a toy Lionel 671 S-2 Turbine Steam train chugging around and around a Christmas tree on Christmas Eve.

As I drove another twenty feet forward in my SUV, I was now closer to where the rocks had fallen from the side of the mountain. Just briefly surveying the scene, I saw at least two boulders blocking the road. Each boulder weighed around eighty to two hundred pounds. At least three of the boulders had hit a tree and knocked it into the road. Police and fire personnel were monitoring the perimeter and keeping everyone safe. And to do the job well, there were two strategically placed Cat 349e Excavators on the scene. The senior road worker said to his junior colleague, “I’m going to bet that there are [going to be] more rock slides like this in the county in this coming week, especially with all the heavy rainfall that we have been having the past two weeks!" The junior colleague responded, "That's true, but I [have] never seen so many come down like this at one time. My truck, coming here, had its rear wheels spin a little bit." The senior road worker continued, "I got me a twelve-inch turkey sandwich with lettuce, tomatoes, black olives, cucumbers, and pepper jack cheese on it." The junior colleague responded, "Man, you gotta stop right there because all I got is a tuna melt sandwich. It was the best I could make before coming here!" After I heard them talking, my belly began to rumble and I could feel sharp hunger pains. I knew that when I got home that night, I would make myself some turkey drumsticks. I was just thinking to myself, I sure did not want to be anywhere nearby when this mountain had its contractions and delivered a precious little rockslide to us motorists situated below its strike zone.

Those construction excavators cleared that pile in about 30 to 45 minutes. I was still listening to my music, so I was not the least bit fazed. The road crews had a Black Decker power saw and cut the downed twenty-foot-tall tree in some five pieces and cleared the roadway in about forty minutes. As soon as the path cleared, the opposing traffic started to come through. When it was my turn to pass by in my SUV, I saw one boulder with jagged edges weighing around three hundred pounds! It looked as if the mountain had just given birth to a baby rock, and now the mountain could rest for another nine months without giving us motorists trouble by dropping her rocky little children to the sides of the road, without any regard about smashing us drivers by dropping her new bundle of joy onto those traveling down below her. I finally, after being cleared by the DOT workers, headed home for the evening.

Anyway, back to the point, Mr. Zax is very soft spoken and usually rides the public transportation bus with about five to six other patients who come in for treatment the day. All the patients that ride on this shuttle all attest to the fact that they feel like second-class citizens when the transportation service just cancels on them, which sometimes makes them miss their counseling sessions and their medical treatments that generally all occur on the same day. If the service cancels on them at the last minute, they usually get a ride from a friend the next day, but they look rough. I remember Mr. Zax came in the next day when he was not picked up by the transportation service. He was sweating profusely, yawning frequently, and his blue and gold WVU T-shirt was drenched. He looked as if he had played four quarters in one of their games. He took off his green baseball cap and it was soaked through and through. He breathed deeply and then stated, "Doc, I'm sure glad to see you today. I was puking several times last night and I'm happy that I won't have to go through that for another day!" I responded, "Man, I'm glad you here too. Let's continue your treatments!" Mr. Zax came back the next week and he was relaxed and calm. He was sporting a fresh set of blue stonewashed denim jeans, new black Converse sneakers, and a freshly pressed gray hoodie that did not have a single piece of lint on it. He was sharp and focused! I love that!

Moving on to issue number two of my CARE model, there may be childcare issues that impede patients from getting to our clinic before we close. Many times, our patients have a newborn baby that no one can take care of for several possible reasons. The grandmother may be in the hospital having chemotherapy treatments or open-heart surgery. The father of the baby may be in prison and cannot be there in the child's life, let alone tend to the baby during the time the mother is coming to our clinic for treatments. Or the father could have run off with another woman. I see all these cases at my clinic at least once a week and I review strategies that a patient may not have thought of to have their child kept safe while they are being clinically evaluated at our clinic.

I am very lucky if a woman with a newborn baby has a husband that is courageous, enough to receive treatment for himself and at the same time has a mild temperament toward his children and decides to be in his child's life. I saw one such couple at the clinic. The man was always with his girlfriend and both were getting treatment, and they brought their child with them. The man, Mr. Jace, always wore a cool-looking black bandanna, thin-rimmed glasses, had a tattoo of a cross on his right forearm; he had an upbeat attitude, what I call an "attitude of gratitude." He did not think anyone owed him anything. He knew that he was at our addiction treatment center by choice—his choice! He had a beautiful baby girl with ocean blue eyes and beautiful blonde hair and such a pretty smile. His girlfriend stood five feet two inches tall and weighed 130 pounds. Mr. Jace was around four inches taller. Ms. Patz, his girlfriend, was also a positive-minded individual and always greeted you with a smile and was grateful to be in our program.

I knocked on the door of the examination room one Wednesday afternoon when it was raining and a brisk 38 degrees outside our clinic. I said, “Good morning, Ms. Patz, how in the world are you doing today?” She began, “Hi, Doc, I’m just glad to be in this program!” I responded, “That’s good, Ms. Patz.” I waved my right hand back and forth at their baby girl, who smiled back at me and started to coo while sitting in the lap of her mother, who was wearing stonewashed blue denim jeans. Even the baby was a fresh breath of air and the perfect little fit for this wonderful couple. The baby giggled and cooed some more, and this was the highlight of my day. No matter how busy the clinic is, at such times, you can take a breather and see the positivity that this clinic is having in the community. The cooing and laughter from the three-month-old baby was the sun that sort of parted the clouds on that rainy day. Mr. Jace remarked, "Me and my girl try to stay positive for our little baby girl." He continued, "Life is what you make it, and we are going to do everything we can to stay clean. Our daughter is our life!" As I listened to his heart with my Littman's cardiology stethoscope as he was perched on the blue examination table with the foot pedestal out, I found even his heart beat was smooth and relaxed, without any skipped beats. Lots of patients get anxiety just from coming to the doctor's office, and you frequently hear skipped heartbeats and irregular cardiac rhythms, as seen in patients that may have a history of atrial fibrillation. But not Mr. Jace. Mr. Jace gives you a firm handshake that does not tremble and he looks you directly in the eye with a gutsy determination like a sailor standing tall outside of a Nimitz warship on a frigid January morning. Even though wind gusts may make the air temperature thirty degrees below zero, the sailor refuses to blink. Mr. Jace's stare was the provenance of pure immutable determination. Mr. Jace loved his newborn baby girl and he told me, "Doc, I'm doing whatever it takes so she doesn't end up like me and my girl. We want better for her—we just got to have better!" I saw that with every muscle fiber in his body, he meant it. His pupils would become dilated, accompanied by simultaneous flaring of his nostrils, whenever he spoke with absolute intention—the intention of having the absolute best for his family.

The next week when the family came to our office, they were going to do something special after their visit to us. Mr. Jace wore a clean gray dress shirt without a single wrinkle in it. I began, "Good morning, Mr. Jace."

He responded, “Good morning, Doc. How’s it going?” I responded, “Very well, and you and the ‘Mrs.’ look very sharp today! What’s the special occasion?” He responded, “Well, Doc, I’ve been waiting a long time... today we are going to take some family photographs.” I responded, “That’s exciting and I’m happy for you.” That gray shirt was absolutely spotless! The girlfriend had a spotless blue blouse and beige khaki pants. It was wonderful seeing them dressed so well, and their baby girl eyed me with a wide grin as if to give her absolute approval.

Three weeks later, they brought in their family photo with them dressed in clothes from the 1930s. It was truly a great photo and that baby of theirs was all smiles. It took them nearly thirty minutes to get that baby to smile just right in that magenta-hued black and white vintage photo.

Now, let us look at number three from the CARE

model. There may be drug-addicted children of the drug-addicted parent that cause the drug-addicted parent grief. I had a thirty-eight-year-old patient that had been addicted to heroin, Oxycontin, and cocaine for around twelve years. She had wavy blond hair and possessed a very affable nature. She stood five feet four inches tall and weighed 205 pounds. Whenever I knocked on the examination room door, she usually jumped off the examination table and said, “Doc, you scared me by that knock on the door, but I like how you see us patients in a timely way!” I responded, “Thanks, Ms. Tee, for your kind words.” She continued, “Must be a busy day. I see you are sweating.” I responded, “Indeed, we have quite a number of patients to help today.” I then pulled out the examination table step and helped her up onto the beige-colored exam table with the oceanic blue carpet below. The room is fifteen feet by ten feet and feels spacious to the patients; plastered on the white walls are posters detailing the damage that different drugs have on different parts of the human body. Ms. Tee then said, "Doc, look at that poster over there!" She had a very sudden elevated pitch in her voice. I looked at the poster for all of five seconds and then I heard it! While looking at the poster, I heard an initially inaudible sob, but then by the time I looked back at Ms. Tee, she was wailing and her eyes were bloodshot red. I rushed out of the room and returned with several Kleenex. She wiped her tears and blew her nose several times. She pointed her finger at one particular poster and said, "That is the one. It is destroying us badly!" I looked over my right shoulder in the direction of the poster and stated, "Is it this one?" She nodded her head in confirmation. I continued, "The methamphetamine poster?" "Yes," she responded and was now crying inconsolably. I asked her, "Ms. Tee, have you ever tried methamphetamine?" "Yes," she responded. She went on to say, "I didn't like it and I didn't use it after that!" I was at least relieved that she was not a long-term methamphetamine user, and her urine drug screens and confirmatory testing corroborated that fact. However, she went on to say, "My son tore up my house last night in a bitter rage!" I ask her what happened. She stated, "My son is a good boy and he used to only smoke weed, but he got with a girl who is a methamphetamine addict who shoots up for days at a time! Doc, you gotta help him and me!" She continued, "When I met his girlfriend the first time, the first thing she said was, 'I get the best high from meth and feel so good!'" Ms. Tee continued, "Doc, I'm so scared. I had a friend who took methamphetamine and died from a severe heart attack. I'm so scared my boy will die from it!" She went on to mention, "I just want my son to stay away from that girl—she's going to get him killed!"

Ms. Tee is from Quinwood, near Marfrance, West Virginia, and this is her daily cross to bear. She weeps uncontrollably whenever she thinks of her son. The thing is, no matter how many times I hear of these parents who are addicted and have children that are addicted, I still get choked up and want to give the parents the best fighting chance I can by getting them sober so they can fight the good fight for their children. Ms. Tee then added, “I’m scared that the meth lab that my son is building will blow up in his face one day.”

I remember when I was working at the Michigan Department of Corrections, I had a patient, Mr. Perkins, who was a chronic methamphetamine user, and when I looked at him for the first time, he had healed third- and fourth-degree burns over 50 percent of his body. He had to get skin grafts from his gluteus maximus to his face, chest, and arms. I asked Mr. Perkins what happened and he responded, “I was shooting up the meth, and the next thing you know, I saw the flames of hell! There was fire as far as my eyes could see, and glass was buried deep in my body!" He was hospitalized for six weeks and was in physical and occupational therapy for about three months afterward. They had to teach him how to walk, eat, and chew his food properly so he would not choke. Parts of his cornea were burned, and he had to have ocular antibiotics for another four months while wearing dark sunglasses to protect his eyes from the sun. I asked if he had any more cravings for methamphetamine. He responded bluntly, "Absolutely not!"

The dynamics of these families are so intricate as generation after generation of families are intertwined with cocaine, methamphetamine, crack, and heroin. Ms. Tee continued, "Doc, you got to talk to our city hall or mayor or something." She had been doing exceptionally well and had not tested positive for any heroin, fentanyl, or Oxycodone, but ever since her son had fallen into methamphetamine, her cravings for her old lifestyle were slowly trying to creep in. But she had been a courageous knight in keeping them at bay.

When I checked back with Ms. Tee three weeks later and asked her how her son was doing, she responded, "At least he is not with his girlfriend and he is looking better for now." Her son's girlfriend was from California, and as a mom, Ms. Tee felt her son was with a girl that lived a very fast and unpredictable lifestyle.

Another patient of mine, Ms. Pax, was raped at the age of 15 and became pregnant with a baby boy. She is in her mid-thirties and stands five feet tall and weighs 180 pounds. She abused methamphetamine to escape the real pain of being violated. Her once baby boy—now 16 years later—stands a towering six foot seven and is addicted to several illicit drugs. When she tries to provide correction, he threatens bodily harm to her and, at his height, he could easily carry through on that promise. Ms. Pax told me that her son says to her, "I don't have to listen to you because you are a druggie!" Tears started to slowly form in her eyes and she said, “Doc, I don’t know what to do!” I told her, “Bring him here. I want to talk with him!” Even if I cannot be a positive male role model for him, I just want to talk with him.

Let us consider number eight from the CARE model. There may be marital stressors. One patient of mine, Mr. Vance, decided to come home early one night after work and, to his surprise, he heard a commotion upstairs where his wife usually slept! Mr. Vance ran to the bedroom to make sure his wife was alright and found her in the very act of infidelity! The stranger that was in Mr. Vance’s bedroom catapulted out of the window, nimbly jumped down the corner gables of the home, leapfrogged over the backyard fence, and was gone! Mr. Vance related this experience to me with tears welling up in his eyes. He went on, “Doc, I was always faithful to her.” I gently patted him on his shoulder and said, “I’m sorry, man!” He continued, “I don’t know what brought this on, Doc." I replied, "Man, these things are hard to prepare for. It's so sudden!" He responded, "I know." Mr. Vance added, "I'm leaving her, Doc!" Quite frankly, it was a challenging situation, and I cannot even begin to imagine how devastating this must have been for Mr. Vance to go through. I continued, "Mr. Vance, I'm going to arrange counseling for you. I think it will do you some good."

A few weeks later, his home was destroyed by a house fire, and he and his wife were now in a homeless shelter. During this interval, they started to become emotionally close. Mr. Vance explained to me four weeks after his wife's affair, "Being in this homeless shelter has given me time to think. I may NOT entirely give up on this marriage!" Mr. Vance was addicted to heroin and opioids for close to 10 years. Through it all he was still a knight that fought to stay clean from drugs while trying to remain on good terms with his wife. When she had this affair, he was stressed out and he related to me, “Doc, she drove me to the brink of abusing heroin again!” And let me tell you something, if he had obtained the wrong type (not that any type of heroin is good, of course, but the wrong type in the sense that this particular street brand could have been laced with carfentanil, a powerful elephant tranquilizer), he might have taken his last ten to twelve breaths before passing out, with death rapidly ensuing.

I encouraged Mr. Vance to take it one day at a time, like when I run up a mountain on a twenty-mile trek for the morning. I do not look up at the mountain and become overwhelmed; rather, I look down at my two feet that are firmly planted on the ground beneath me and become ferociously determined that the only direction I am going to go is forward from this current vantage point. Though my current vantage point is in the valley, once I move forward, that direction will only naturally propel me up through the valley and up and over those hills of rocks that are looking down on me!

Another patient of mine, Ms. Lux, had been a heroin and crack addict for twelve years. One time, she shot up crystal methamphetamine, and later said to me, “Doc, that is something I will never, ever do again in my life!” I asked her, “Why is that?” She responded, “Well, Doc, when I shot that crystal meth into my arm, you won’t believe what I saw!” I asked her, “What did you see?” She responded, “Doc, after I shot up, I saw the Devil, and he stood around seven feet tall and had long fingers about a foot long, and he was running after me fast. He was twirling his tongue out at me in order to trip me as I was running away from him!” I asked her, “What prevented the Devil from getting you?” She responded, “My mother is a praying woman and pastor, and something told her to pray at the same time that I was having this battle with the Devil. Then, suddenly, he turned around and ran right off in the opposite direction." The Devil she described said to her while she was high on methamphetamine, "I'm going to drag you to hell like I did your sister!" So, I asked her about her sister and she confirmed that her sister had died of an opiate overdose several years earlier. On top of this, she ran with the top drug kingpins in the state and witnessed one individual having a gun placed two inches from his head and the trigger being pulled, with his brains exploding onto the ground along with the entire half of his face in a lake of blood. She said, "Doc, I could not cry!" I responded, "A person was just shot point blank in the head and you did not cry. WHY?" She responded, "Because if I even blinked, he was going to turn the gun on me and shoot me in the head!" To which I responded, "Oh, man!"

Ms. Lux, too, has a son that is now an opiate addict. She confided in me that she had to put him out of the house for reasons of her recovery from drug addiction and her personal safety. For some reason, all these mothers have sons that are over six feet four inches tall. Once these sons attain such a physical stature, they are often physically dominating in the household, especially where no father is around. Ms. Lux said, “I love my son, but it is what it is. This is MY recovery and I just can't have NO ONE get in the way of MY recovery right now. I just can’t!” I admired her pugnacious approach to her recovery. She continued, “I got to be strong for me first, then I can help him later after I am FULLY recovered.” She was kicking her leg back and forth against the trays of the examination table while her head was lowered, and her eyes alternated between the floor and looking deeply into mine. She was a knight in that she was going to War, that is, she was going to “Wage A Resistance”—a resistance against anything or anyone that would impede her recovery from opiate addiction. She also separated from her husband, who was abusing cocaine, heroin, and opiates. She stated, “Doc, I’m just going to do whatever it takes and separate from anyone who is going to drag me down!” She was dressed in light blue denim jeans and a white blouse, with her long nails painted in pink. Whenever she spoke with such fierce intention, she would either dig her nails into the beige exam chair five times or fold her arms with clenched fists. Her urine drug tests were clean. She meant business and was not only “talking the talk” at our center but also “letting her walk” back up her talk. Ms. Lux always had a glassy stare with sunken in eyes and moistened lips. I knew she was serious and I would fight with her for a complete recovery. When she spoke, it was not just from the lips, it was from somewhere deep below near her diaphragm, and her neck muscles would vibrate forcefully when she spoke. Her forehead glistened from the beads of sweat that had accumulated atop her brow and would drop to the sides of her face and onto the blue carpet below. When she spoke, you felt every molecule of your soul listening to what she was saying to you. She had black eyes that would stare right into your soul as every word she spoke was rich in content. She spoke with deep revelation when she talked of distancing herself from family members that would drag her backward on her road to recovery from crack and heroin addiction.

Another patient, Ms. Atkins, had herself been a long-term abuser of opiates and benzodiazepines, and I educated her on the dangers of taking an opiate with Xanax as it causes you to stop breathing by interfering with the area of the brain stem that controls breathing. Ms. Atkins was jolted back into reality when a friend she grew up with overdosed. "What's happening today, Ms. Atkins?" I began. Ms. Atkins is a petite five-foot-two woman around 110 pounds, and has the longest eyelashes I have ever seen. She has streaked blond hair, and whenever she speaks, she nods her head forward to give her words extra meaning. She has red freckles and generally holds her head at an angle when she converses with our staff. She began, “My best friend is on a ventilator and his blood pressure was 200 over 120!” She continued, “I don’t know what to do!” I saw her one week later in the clinic and she stated, “The doctors tried Narcan and got no response from my friend.” She continued, “They have turned off the respirator and have pronounced him dead.” Tears meanwhile were welling up in her eyes, and I handed her several tissues to wipe her tears and blow her nose. She continued, “He was only thirty-one and left behind a five-year-old and a thirteen-year-old. In his system they found Xanax, Oxycontin, and crystal methamphetamine.” I give her my condolences and allowed her to have some private time to herself, and then she wept inconsolably. However, this same week, she herself tested positive for opiates and simultaneous benzodiazepines. I continued to instruct her on the dangers of combining these two medications. She informed me, “Doc, my nerves are shattered. I’m sorry.”

Let us move on to my next patient. Ms. Peaches was on heroin and had abused opiates for the past 10 years. She now has a twenty-one-year-old daughter who is eight months pregnant and is shooting crack cocaine, crystal methamphetamine, and heroin into her veins. Ms. Peaches said to me, “Doc, I am just devastated. I just can’t continue to let my daughter continue on like this!” I responded, “Then Ms. Peaches, what do you think you are going to do?” She said, “I am going to call Child Protective Services and go through the legal process to get sole custody of my grandbaby!” Now that is a super intelligent thing to do. She does not want her grandchild to end up in the foster care system. I do not want to refer to any child that is already in the foster care system as “lost” because I feel they are worth more than that term.

Numerous grandparents have had to raise their grandchildren because their child is addicted to crack, heroin, and methamphetamine. I constantly struggle to come up with solutions for this population. Many grandparents tell me, "Dr. Alexis, I thought I would have it easy and just relax, but now lately I am faced with the total care of my grandson and granddaughter."

Let us look at issue number four of the CARE model. There may be a child that recently died who belonged to the person with an opiate use disorder (OUD). One of my patients, Ms. Blanchard, had just lost a son to brain cancer. She had been struggling with heroin and pain pills for years. She was a blond-haired woman standing five foot five who always spoke softly. Her first husband used to violently assault her and had fractured several bones in her face. She had also sustained a hemorrhage in the brain because of this brutal man's random assaults, and had to spend close to a month in the hospital to undergo multiple facial reconstructive surgeries! As a result, she possessed an inner fire in her spirit. She would look you directly in the eye whenever she spoke. Though she would still speak softly, she would let you know what she expected out of her treatment sessions. She was good at attending her counseling sessions that dealt with the triggers associated with relapse. She relapsed on cocaine and pain pills after losing her son to brain cancer. I remember like it was yesterday. Around three months earlier, she had brought her son to our office one day. Her son wore a slight smile and did not seem to have a care in the world. The next time I heard from her, she was at his bedside and he was valiantly fighting cancer. He fought courageously, but despite all the medical treatments, he passed away. How sad. I could feel the tears starting to sting my eyes. I reviewed the medical records of her son and was so saddened.

Since then, she has come back to our clinic and has

been drug-free for the past thirty days, and I am extremely proud of her. She brought me a red and green coffee mug, which she had gift-wrapped, and a Christmas card. She is amazing! She is a courageous knight that stood tall despite the loss of her son from a brain tumor and came back to our clinic despite her own battles with cocaine and pain pills. Her son was an even bigger knight. Having to battle autism and a malignant brain tumor, he was a warrior knight. He was fighting two wars at once. He fought with a double-edged sword! One side of the sword was faith and the other side was perseverance. He did not lose this battle! He, in fact, won it! God has made him an eternal knight and no disease or pain can touch him, and he stands tall at the side of the King of Kings and the Lord of Lords. The Great I AM.

I have already discussed issue number 5, custody battles that a parent has with their ex-spouse. So now let us look at CARE model number 6, coexisting mental health issues with a patient's drug addiction. One of my patients was very anxious and suffered from major depressive disorder after years of physical abuse by her boyfriend, and she was very tearful each time I saw her. She was a 120-pound, five-foot-tall petite woman and was wearing blue jeans and a red and green sweater as it was close to Christmas. She asked me, "Doc, what do I need to do to make everything right?" Tears were falling from her ocean blue eyes, making their way down the side of her high cheekbones that gently curved inwardly to her lower jaw. I responded, "Ms. Davis, I will walk you through this process one day at a time." I then asked her, "Are you still in this abusive relationship?" She responded, "No." I was glad for this because many women end up with severe physical injuries or even dead before they can make their escape. She had just made the first and best choice in creating some degree of separation from this abuser.

Let us again revisit the stats related to opioid use. There are 2.3 million people addicted to opioids. Around twelve million have misused opioids in the past twelve months alone! One hundred people die daily from opioid abuse or one person every twelve minutes. Thirty-six million people are addicted to opioids worldwide. What has caused this? Well... Oxycodone prescription writing surged from 76 million in 1991 to 210 million in 2013 when pharmaceutical companies claimed that their pain medications were not addictive, when they were. Emergency Department visits related to overdoses increased from 145,000 in 2004 to 310,000 in 2008. In 2002, 12,000 people died from opioids, and by 2015, there was a near threefold increase as 33,000 people had died. In 1973, there were 328,600 arrests for drug law violation, according to the FBI, and in 2016, that number skyrocketed to 1,572,579. Recently, FDA approved a once-a-month subcutaneous injection for opioid use disorder. This medication is Sublocade, which shows promise in helping patients take their medication in a scheduled fashion with less risk of diversion to the drug, and with less chance of them forgetting to take their medication.

I asked Ms. Davis about her hobbies, and she mentioned that she liked to read as it took her mind away from the pain. A week later, I bought her a book just so she could have some leverage in equipping herself for success over her prior pain. I do not expect for her emotional pain to be vanquished in a day, week, month, or even a year. Rather, I am creating a lifestyle of mental and cognitive change on a weekly basis when I see her. Number one, I teach her to War, "wage a resistance," against her fears by not blaming herself for those years of physical abuse that led to her finding an escape via the seducing pink crystal of crack and crystal methamphetamine. She was never weak but was a knight in facing a monster that physically abused her. Number two, she also had a WHY, "wisdom holding you." Sometimes, it feels that life is so harsh and unforgiving that there is no ground beneath you. That is, when you must go into BEAST ("beholding endless aspirations while standing tall") mode to know that you will fight those inner voices that say you are not strong and life was meant to be this way. The brain's circuitry naturally tends to follow the path of least resistance. In such instances, you have to say out loud that your recovery from drugs or departure from abusive relationships is intended to preserve the very first relationship, that is, the relationship of fierce dedication to your mind's piece of mental peace. When I talk about a "mind piece," I am referring to a portion of your mind that you reserve for yourself that is full of tranquility, which will serve you well both now and later. However, will obtaining that peace come easy? Of course not! That is why you must be vigilant to mentally fight all negative influences that will speak to your mind throughout the day. As stated in 2 Corinthians 10:5, "Casting down imaginations, and every high thing that exalts itself against the knowledge of God, and bringing into captivity every thought to the obedience of Christ." All of us get thoughts that we wrestle with, like should we take an extra cupcake on the relative innocuous side of things, all the way to should I buy that gram of heroin, as in the case of those with opioid use disorder. You must have the desire to be successful by separating that piece of your mind that will only take your inner peace away.

Anyway, the Christmas blues can be a challenge, mentally and emotionally, for many of my patients. They live in poverty and many just do not have a support system. Their families feel that it is a huge stigma even to acknowledge their existence, and my patients feel the sting of this daily. There is often no one to invite them home for a warm meal, and they are, literally, left to fend for themselves. Will I look at these blessed souls and hear them pour their hearts out and just walk away? Hell no! I will take their hand and we will pray in the name of Jesus that he will bring peace and resolution to their problem. Does this work? Yes! I had one patient that wanted more working hours at his job for a trucking company. One week after we prayed and believed, he reported to me that his work hours had went up by another 35 hours for that one week! Amazing! Another gentleman had a job at a local fast food joint that was giving him, at best, sporadic work hours, around twenty-four hours weekly, at $10 per hour. About two weeks after I prayed with my patient, he was offered a job as an electrician at a nuclear power plant paying $30/hour, with forty to fifty hours guaranteed, and with breakfast and lunch covered! Was this a coincidence? Certainly not. I believe that prayer works and the power of Jesus Christ is what makes all the difference! Another patient, a coal miner, was working forty hours a week, and I asked, “Peter, how is work coming along in the mines?” He responded, “Well, Doc, it’s ok, but I need more hours as I got a wife and three kids to support!” I said, “Peter, would you like to pray? It won’t hurt at all.” Peter responded, “Of course, Doc, let’s do this!” I prayed for him, and three weeks later, he got a job promotion to director of the mines, which came with an increase to his hourly pay of $25, and an increase of his work hours by an additional thirty hours weekly!!! Again, is this coincidence? Of course not. Another woman had a son that was abusing the monstrous seducing pink crystal methamphetamine and she requested prayer. We prayed, and two weeks later when I asked her how her son was doing, she reported through tears that he was not abusing crystal methamphetamine anymore and was not interacting with the girlfriend that had tried to get him to take more of this vile substance. I felt tears burning my eyes as she told me this.

I was profoundly transformed by the power of prayer for my fellow human beings that connects us to the ultimate source—God. These depressed patients look to me for answers, and I reassure them that just because today looks limited in its options for them, does not mean that tomorrow will be the exact replica of such misery. The possibilities are endless for a positive outcome, but they must first believe that positive things are in their immediate reach. Once they realize this, they can reach and undoubtedly RULE—“realm of unlimited and lustrous eminence”—their lives for the Good and never be vanquished as a dying knight. But rather, they can conquer and crush the seducing pink crystal as a victorious knight. Another patient of mine, Mr. Bowne remarked, “I’m so happy today!” I asked Mr. Bowne, “Why is that?” He continued, “Doc, I just got my tax refund of $4,000 today, and prior to being in your program, this would have all been spent on drugs!" I responded, "I'm so happy for you, Mr. Bowne!" He continued, "I purchased a Pontiac Grand Am instead and, boy, is she a beauty!" I was truly pleased with Mr. Bowne. What have all the patients of mine that I have described done that played a role in their success? They created a PICTURE, "painting into cognition the ultimate reality to embrace." In painting, on the white canvas of their minds, they are mentally designing the innate strategies that will help them in avoiding the negative crowd they once associated with. They are firmly implanting those strategies into their mind-set as their reality. This must be the reality that they embrace with their physical actions. They can fool us by saying all the right things in counseling or when they see me during their visit to the physician's office. But their choice of not going to that particular New Year's party where the seducing pink crystal methamphetamine is present along with crack, cocaine, Oxycodone, Roxicet, and Opanas is exactly the embrace that I teach and intimately foster with each of my patients I see weekly, who number in the hundreds. One patient of mine, for New Year's day 2018, did not go out to the party where her friends typically hang out. The music was blaring at that home and was just as seductive as the devilish seducing pink crystal itself. The music draws you in to sit down and mingle in the environment of crystal methamphetamine, cocaine, Oxycontin, LSD—the cesspool chamber of death! She told me that she learned from people who went to the party that there were illicit filthy drugs of all sorts—heroin, crack, cocaine, LSD, ecstasy. She also said, "And, Doc, they were FREE too!" But let us analyze that statement for just a second. These same drugs that 1) get you hooked and make you illicitly sell your body; 2) cause you to rip off your mother; 3) make you take people hostage at gunpoint; 4) cause you to develop invasive MRSA flesh-eating bacterial infections; 5) infect you with HIV and hepatitis C, from filthy needles; 6) give you heart attacks by making the blood vessel walls of your heart literally explode; 7) make you hemorrhage in your brain; 8) rot away your teeth; 9) make cauliflower-shaped bacterial formations on your heart valves (cardiac abscess); and 10) lead you to abandon your children, leaving them home alone—is that the freedom that you really want? I do not think any of us want to be "FREE" like that!

If you examine it closely, it is the embrace that is the MASTER GLUE that holds my PICTURE paradigm together. To embrace something is to firmly yet endearingly hold something close to one's body, soul, and spirit. You will do whatever it takes to embrace recovery from illicit drugs for your home, your children, your mind, and your very survival. Then and only then is the one time that you will be limitless in your freedom.

God Bless you all in Jesus's name. Amen.

Chapter Three

Prebiotics, the true cure

Most medical Experts will tell you about the benefits of Probiotics as the foundation to Optimum Gut Health. They will also tell you that this also plays a critical role in the link between an enhanced immune system. The one thing that has not been mentioned is something called PREBIOTICS, which is totally different from PROBIOTICS. Without PREBIOTICS, you will not achieve the REAL results of gut health, Mental Health Optimization or an enhanced Immune system that you are desperately in search of. Let us for a moment understand what Prebiotics are. Prebiotics are types of dietary fiber that feed the Good bacteria in your gut. The Good Bacteria in your gut - (You guessed right are the Probiotics). However, Probiotics are USELESS without their partner in crime - that is PREBIOTICS! There are two Primary Prebiotics that your body must have. There's Inulin and Oligofructose. The Left Side of your colon prefers Inulin and the Right side actually prefers oligofructose. These Prebiotics reduce bloating, indigestion and Prebiotics are a source of soluble fiber. Now next you may be asking what foods are Prebiotics? Great Question! Apples, Jerusalem Artichokes, Leeks, Asparagus, Garlic, Onion, Jicama, Barley, Konjac, Cabbage, Bananas, Oats, Flaxseeds, Lentils. This is the short list! If you don't feel energetic, light on your feet, less cognitively alert than you HAVE a deficiency OF PREBIOTICS. I had a patient that was around 40 years of age and I visited him at his group home. We will call him Andrew (Not his real name). One thing that I remember about Andrew was his Absolute Love Affair with Apples. He would eat at least 10 apples a day. You simply could not pry an Apple out of Andrew's Hand or risk being punched in the face suddenly! It was like his Wife or something. He would even look at his Apple and talk to it, then smile at it, kiss it then devour it voraciously. If you dare talk to him at him while he was literally talking to his Apple he would roll his eyes at you and then immediately place his attention back to his First Love - The Beloved Apple. While the majority of patient's at this Special Needs Group home suffered from Constipation and other Gut issues like hemorrhoids from having to push so hard from constipated stool - that was NEVER an issue for Andrew. If anything, Andrew had Phenomenal Bowel movements! When we call out for Andrew - "Hello Andrew where are you?" We looked at each other in bewilderment. He wasn't playing pool with the other clients and he wasn't watching TV in the Entertainment room. We would be left scratching our heads. Andrew responded - "Silly Goose I'm in the bathroom!" One thing is that he would never flush the toilet as he forgot to do the most mundane of tasks. This resulted in Staff quite frequently SEEING firsthand the WONDERFUL effects that the One Prebiotic that I've mentioned above -namely Apples had on his Bowel Movements! Another way to relieve constipation the NATURAL way without all those pesky medications is to Engage in a campaign of I.F. That is Intermittent Fasting. Let us say for example that you have your last meal of the day at 9 P.M. I strongly suggest that you eat your next meal at 4 P.M. the next afternoon. That is a 18 to 19 hour fast. In between, you can take some Green Tea with ginger roots. The Green tea has natural anxiety relieving properties and the ginger will naturally relieve any nausea that you may initially experience from prolonged periods of fasting. To keep yourself mentally sharp while fasting - to that cup of green tea that you are holding in your hand right now I would sprinkle one teaspoon of turmeric in it. The Turmeric will help in fight joint arthritis and offers additional protection of cancer. The Turmeric can also be protective against Alzheimer's Disease. If you are really feeling motivated at this very moment then you can add some Apple Cider Vinegar to that Green Tea in order to add some Prebiotics to the hot cup of Health and Wellness. You will find that this Intermittent Fasting with one to two miles of walking per day you will have a natural relief of bowel movements. I have other natural constipation relief measures available upon individual consultation. The Blue Zones of The World which are renowned for its people living well pass 100 years of age do form of this Intermittent fasting. Let's look at Okinawa, Japan. They practice the art of hara hachi bu - which is to literally eat until 80% full. Here in The Americas we eat until we are 100% full. But by that time it's already too late. I started practicing hara hachi bu several years ago and I initially was hungry for the first few days like 2 or 3 at the most but by the 4th day, my body totally got it! It takes around a half hour for your brain to receive the neurological signaling from your GI Tract that you are full. Once you feel satisfied, that is your

TRUE full set point. You don't have to eat until you are stuffed. Don't clean your plate! There is also another way to genetically enable yourself to also LIVE LONGER. I do this activity on Friday's, Saturday's and Sunday's and if you join my MASTERCLASS WEEKENDS IN PERSON, I will train you how.

ALSO DO YOU SUFFER FROM SINUSITIS, RHEUMATOID ARTHRITIS, FIBROMYALGIA, ECZEMA, PSORIASIS, ACNE, HYPOTHYROID, DEPRESSION, ADHD, ANXIETY? There may be a Deficient amount of Prebiotics in your diet!

Prebiotics produce short chain fatty acids (SCFA's) like Butyrate, Acetate, Propionic and valerate. These SCFA's prevent Colon cancer in several ways. Reduction of the colon's pH. Bifidobacteria and lactobacilli are the good bacteria that reduce the pH in the colon by the production of lactic acid. These lactic acid producing bacteria also manufacture butyrate. Increased Butyrate Levels are linked to cellular death of cancer cells! Probiotics also regulate glucose metabolism and blood pressure and Lowers triglyceride levels. How much Prebiotics then should I be consuming on a daily basis?

That's a Great Question and I'm so glad that you asked! You should generally consume at least 5 grams of prebiotics daily. Do you want a power breakfast loaded in Prebiotics? Have some Oatmeal with Blueberries and sprinkle some Flax seeds in your Oats. Don't forget to add some apples to your morning Oatmeal. With this have an Apple- Cinammon/Bananna Nut -Asparagus Muffin with some warm Butter drizzling down the sides of that Bad Boy! Bite, Lick Ingest and Feast your Gut to Health and Wellness! I will give you Delicious Lunch and Dinner Recipes ONLY with ONE on ONE Consultations at www.medicalwellness.blog.

I offer one-on-one master classes on weekends so that you too can be a courageous knight, and not let any pink seducing crystal stand in your way to obtaining success. Please go to www.medicalwellness.blog to check it out!

Addendum One

THE SEDUCTIVE PINK CRYSTAL

[The five MUST Say Things…]

The five must say things to your child that you may not be able to see again as a drug-addicted mother as you only have 15 minutes to say it afterwards by the 16th minute you will not be able to speak to your 10-year-old son again. Also, you may not be able to see your son ever again after 48 hours as he has just been diagnosed with Terminal Brain Cancer. The reason that you cannot talk to your son after the 15th minute is that he has immediately become unconscious after chemotherapy and he has died at 48 hours, which is the reason you WILL NEVER see him again.

The FIVE MUST things to say, firstly, is that you love him. You must reaffirm this on a constant basis. While saying that you love him you must hold his arm so it

"LOCKS IN" The fact that you really mean it. It is only superficial until you do this. It shows your child that you are locked in the battle to fight up until the very last minute.

Secondly, you EDUCATE your child that you have a chronic disease with your drug addiction. Just like HTN, Diabetes or Asthma, you educate your child that just like they have the disease of cancer you too have a disease and let your child know that you and your child are in the fight together battling something that's intense for the BOTH of you. This makes your child feel that he/she is not alone in this challenge that they are going through.

Thirdly, educate them that you are undergoing treatments for your disease and that they are going to get treatment for their disease so AGAIN your child does not feel forsaken. Let your child know that you are with them. This forms an INNER spiritual Bond with your child that will draw the two of you even closer at this time.

Fourthly, educate your child that you will be more productive and you can and WILL do more of the things your child wants to do while spending less time in drug seeking behaviors - thereby even further strengthening the parent-child bond during this CRITICAL time period.

Lastly, ask your child if they have any questions and if they do – answer them! Give them a hug and tell them that you love them! These are the five MUST SAY things that you MUST communicate to your child!

Addendum Two

THE SEDUCTIVE PINK CRYSTAL

[Hell Hath No Fury]

There was a 35-year-old affable Heroin and Crystal Methamphetamine addict. He related to me that he overdosed on Crystal Methamphetamine and he then fell down into this deep pit. It was so dark that you could cut the darkness with a knife. It also started to get EXTREMELY HOT. When my patient opened his eyes, he could clearly see walls of fire 100 feet high and he himself was in a mega lake of fire! It was as hot as molten lava this went on for day after day and night after night for 30 days as he was in a coma! He relates to me as his physician and felt very comfortable sharing the whole details of what happened to him without any reservation at all. He remembers crying out "Jesus if you are real - please get me out of this place!" He also told me that for

30 days and 30 nights straight that second after second his skin painfully melted off of his body and only his skeleton remained! His skin would then come back on the skeletal frame just to be melted off once again. He said it was the most traumatizing event of his life! As he cried out to the Lord Jesus he remembered all the times that he did go to church as a young child with his parents but as he grew older did not see the importance of staying faithful to the Lord Jesus and so he strayed away. He refused to even give the Lord Jesus one hour in prayer let alone go to church for one hour per week. So when he cried out to the Lord again All of a sudden the most brilliant and bright light shone there in Hell at least one-thousand times brighter than looking at the sun face on and then suddenly a booming dominating voice said "John you have NOT been Faithful to me!" Suppose I was not faithful to you and left you in these flames of Hell - how would you feel? Then slowly he felt his soul being lifted out of that

dreadful, dark and fiery hot place. The flames now not being able to tear the flesh off his body and render him a skeleton. John vowed to Jesus that he would go to church EVERY Sunday and would not be LUKEWARM in his relationship any longer with Jesus Christ. Shortly thereafter, he woke up in his ICU bed with tubes going down his throat and all kinds of IV's in his arms. The ICU physician seen John's eyes open up WIDE! The ICU team performed some quick preliminary tests before taking the breathing tube out of John's mouth. Later that evening he was able to eat his first real meal in 30 days and he was too ashamed to tell this story because he was afraid of what others would think. It took him the utmost courage to tell me even this much of his story.

References

1) 6 Ancient Cultures and their Obsession with Crystals- Matt Caron, Sivana East.

2) Different Uses Of Crystals - Lucy Dale.

3) Steve Cushing: 24 th *Marathon des Sables- A* Competitors tale. Leicester UK, Matador 2010.

4) Guy Giaoui, Foued Berahou:*Ultramarathon Stage Racing- From* our experience *of* The *Marathon des Sables, The TransAg*; *and* other races- *A Practical Guide.* ST -Genest-Malifaux, Raidlight 2008.

5) Mark Hines- *The Marathon des Sables- Seven Days in The Sahara*-enduring *The Toughest footrace on Earth.* London, Health Body Publishing 2007.

6) Monika Nicolle:*Histoire* d'un *Marathon des Sables- 245 Kilometres dans le desert.* Paris, Editions de l'une 2010.

7) Eddy Poirier: *Vaincre soi-meme:Marathon des Sables! Toute une histoire* [S.I.] Glob. 2009.

8) Pierre - Emmanuel Bastion: *Regard sur le Marathon des Sables*:2004/06 Biarritz, SAI 2007.

9) Hew -Butler, Tamara; Ayus J. Carlos; Kips, Courtney; Maughan, Ronald J; Mettler, Samuel:Meeuwise, Willem H; Page, Anthony J; Reid, Stephen A; Rehrer, Nancy J et. al 92008) "Statement of the Second International Exercise Associated Hyponatremia Consensus Development Conference, New Zealand, 2007." *Clinical Journal of Sport Medicine*. 18 (2):111-21.

10) Noakes, T. *Waterlogged: The Serious Problem of* over hydration *in Endurance Sports*. Human Kinetics, 2012.

11) Siegel AJ, Verbalis JG, Clement S, et al. Hyponatremia in Marathon runners due to Inappropriate arginine vasopressin secretion. Am. J. Med. 2007; 120:461.e11.

12) Drogue HJ, Madias NE. Hyponatremia. *New England Journal* Of *Medicine* 2000;342:1581.

13) Crack overdose:How much amount of Crack to OD? Addiction Blog.

14) These 15 medications can cause a False Positive on Drug Tests. Good Rx Prescription Savings Blog.

15) 20 amazing Benefits of Sage Herb for skin, Hair and Health. Vineetha.

16) Which country would be hardest to invade? *Independent* May 01 2015.

17) NIH- NIDA - "Methamphetamine". 02/2017.

18) NIH - NIDA "Mind Over Matter:Methamphetamine" 10/27/2017.

19) Michael Jordan Didn't make Varsity- At First- *Newsweek*. 10/17/2015.

20) 12 foods with more Vitamin C than Oranges. - Christine Mattheis 12/30/2012.

21) 11 Amazing Benefits of Pineapples- Organicfacts.net

22)Tuberculosis Fact Sheets Centers For Disease Control & Prevention 10/28/2011.

23) "A Slow heartbeat in Athletes is not so Funny" - *Science NEWS* 05/21/2014.

24) Sick Sinus Syndrome : Clinical Manifestations, Diagnosis and Evaluation - Munther K. Homoud M.D. Up To Date.

25) Vagal Maneuvers Daniel Frisch M.D. Up To Date 10/30/2017.

26) Menopausal Hot Flashes - Richard canteen et al Up To Date 11/21/2017.

Made in United States
North Haven, CT
04 November 2026

21772726R00157